Fast & Feast

90 Weight Loss Recipes to Eat In Between Fasts

I0843299

© **Copyright 2018 - All rights reserved.**

The contents of this book may not be reproduced, duplicated or transmitted without direct written permission from the author.

Under no circumstances will any legal responsibility or blame be held against the publisher for any reparation, damages, or monetary loss due to the information herein, either directly or indirectly.

Legal Notice:

This book is copyright protected. This is only for personal use. You cannot amend, distribute, sell, use, quote or paraphrase any part of the content within this book without the consent of the author.

Disclaimer Notice:

Please note the information contained within this document is for educational and entertainment purposes only. Every attempt has been made to provide accurate, up to date and complete, reliable information. No warranties of any kind are expressed or implied. Readers acknowledge that the author is not engaging in the rendering of legal, financial, medical or professional advice. The content of this book has been derived from various sources. Please consult a licensed professional before attempting any techniques outlined in this book.

By reading this document, the reader agrees that under no circumstances is the author responsible for any losses, direct or indirect, which are incurred as a result of the use of information contained within this document, including, but not limited to, —errors, omissions, or inaccuracies.

Table of Contents

40.   Extra-Lean Burger and Salad

41.   Cowboy Beef

42.   Cream of Chicken Soup

43.   Pan Fried Italian Chicken Thighs

44.   Chicken and Vegetable Curry

45.   Warm Chicken Salad

46.   Chicken and Vegetable Balti

47.   Chicken Butternut Chili

48.   Spicy Chicken and Spelt Salad

49.   Spicy Cajun Chicken Quinoa

50.   Moroccan Chicken & Lentils

51.   Sweet Potato & Chicken with Gravy

52.   Five Spice Chicken Wings

53.   Mango Chicken Tacos

54.   Gingered Chutney Chicken

55.   Sesame Ginger Turkey Wraps

56.   Turkey and Avocado Lettuce Cups

57.   Turkey-Carrot Roll-Up

58.   Pasta with Turkey and Broccoli

59.   Amaranth Fish Sticks

60.   Summer Garden Fish Tacos

61.   Crisp Mashed Potato Fish Cakes

Chapter Three: Occasional Treats

Complementary Book

Thank you for buying my book! If you haven't already, make sure you pick up a copy of my first book:

Intermittent Fasting: A Beginner's Guide to Losing Body Fat with Intermittent Fasting (21 Day Ritual)

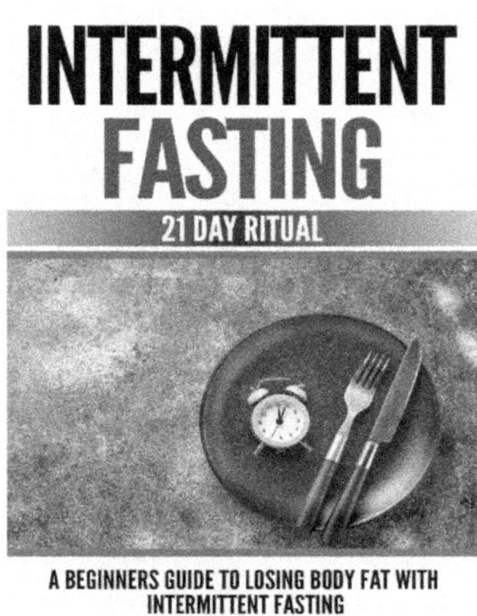

You can get the book by **clicking here:** https://amzn.to/2CTKFMr

The reason I recommend you get the first book is because it teaches you how to intermittent fast. In my opinion, you should *only* be learning what to eat in between your fasts after you've already learned how to fast in the first place! So if you haven't already, make sure to pick up a copy and then come back to this one once you've finished!

Introduction

I want to thank you for buying this book 'Intermittent Fasting: *Fast & Feast: 90 Weight Loss Recipes to Eat In Between Fasts*' and I hope you will find it interesting and useful.

The world is rapidly changing and, if you do not change accordingly, you will fall behind and suffer. It is necessary to keep on with the competition in this dog eat dog world. The ever-growing competition has reached almost all sections of human life and it should not come as a surprise that even basic things such as fitness and health have become competitive.

Everyone wants to stay fit, look attractive and be healthy. However, due to hectic schedules and unhealthy lifestyle, it has become extremely difficult to maintain a good body. Not many of us have the time and resources that are crucial to develop our bodies in this way. You may manage to find time for exercise but maintaining a healthy diet still remains a difficult task. But thanks to research, experiences and trials of many others with a similar dilemma, many new and old diets have surfaced and resurfaced. These diets have revolutionized the fitness world and have brought in the much-awaited necessary changes.

Although there are many diets that fall under the above category, one diet plan is still miles ahead of them. Intermittent fasting is an old form of diet that has once again become extremely popular thanks to its convenience, adaptability and various benefits. It is extremely easy to follow and leads to long lasting results.

Intermittent fasting is not a new method of dieting. In fact, people have been doing it since the beginning of time. Certain fasts such as the Ramadan fast, Lent, etc. have been practiced since ancient times. These fasts, though based on beliefs and religions, are still forms of intermittent fasts and have similar positive effects as well. Intermittent fasting basically means eating at particular times during the day and fasting for the remaining time. So, for instance, if you have your breakfast at 8:00 a.m., you are supposed to fast until 8:00 p.m. The fasting period allows your body a resting period and leads to weight loss, glucose regulation and various other benefits.

There exist a variety of intermittent fasts. Some of them are easy to do while some are quite difficult for beginners. Regardless of the ease of an intermittent fast, it can still be one of the most difficult things you ever do if you have never fasted before. You need to regulate your diet cycle, which can be quite a task for many. Yet, it can't be compared to the grueling fact that you need to go 'hungry' for 8-10-12 or even more hours of the day. Eating one or two meals per day and going 'hungry' for the rest is especially difficult for people with busy schedules who are often accustomed to eating anything they find whenever they get the time. Such people avoid doing intermittent fasting because they believe that they cannot stick to the diet or will go hungry.

The popular notion that you need to eat drab and boring diet food while fasting intermittently is a myth. Many books on intermittent fasting are available online, almost all of them fail to mention the above fact. Yes, you can have tasty yet healthy food while you practice intermittent fasting. To make your job easy, here is a book of lip smacking healthy recipes that we have compiled with a plethora of recipes that you can cook at home and eat while you are on an intermittent fast.

Fast & Feast – 90 Weight Loss Recipes to Eat In Between Fasts is a well-researched book that has every possible recipe that you could try out while you are on an intermittent fast. These delicious, easy to make and quick recipes will give you the perfect results that you are looking for with your fast.

All the recipes given in this book are tried tested and tasted and are quite flexible as well. If you do not like an ingredient or believe that a recipe can pop more with the addition of certain ingredients, you can adjust the recipe according to your taste. However, try to keep the nutrients and calorific value of the recipe intact.

A cookbook can make or break a diet, and you can be rest assured, this book one will definitely make yours. I want to thank you once again for choosing this book, let's get started.

Chapter One: Breakfast Recipes

1. Avocado and Mango Green Tea Smoothie

Serves: 2

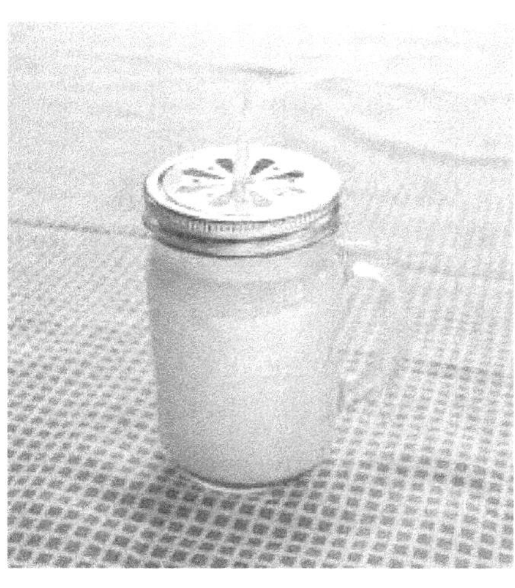

Ingredients:

- 2 cups green tea
- 1 medium avocado, peeled, pitted, cubed
- 1 tbsp coconut oil
- 2 cups mango chunks
- 2 cups spinach, torn
- A pinch of sea salt
- Stevia to taste (optional)

Method:

1. Add all the ingredients in a blender and blend until smooth.
2. Pour into glasses and serve.

2. Green Smoothie

Serves: 2

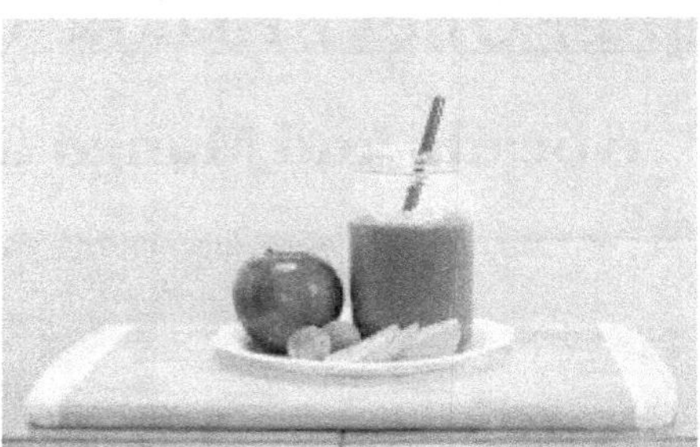

Ingredients:

- 2 avocados, peeled, pitted, cubed
- ½ cup blueberries
- 2 tbsp chia seeds
- 2 cups coconut milk
- 2 cups chard, spinach or kale, discard hard stems and ribs, torn

Method:

1. Add all the ingredients in a blender and blend until smooth.
2. Pour into glasses and serve.

3. Weight Loss Smoothie

Serves: 2

Ingredients:

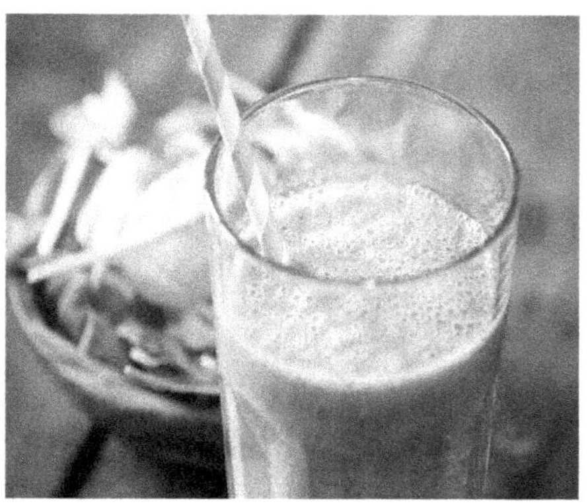

- 2 cups water
- 1 medium avocado, peeled, chopped
- 1 cup blueberries
- 2 tbsp chia seeds
- 1 tbsp coconut oil
- ½ tsp cinnamon powder
- Stevia to taste (optional)

Method:

1. Add all the ingredients in a blender and blend until smooth.
2. Pour into glasses and serve.

4. Chocolate Oatmeal Smoothie

Serves: 2

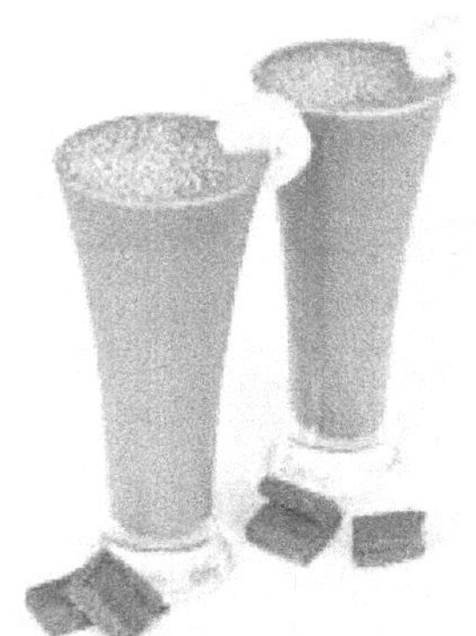

Ingredients:

- ½ cup steel cut oats
- 4 tbsp unsweetened cocoa powder
- Stevia to taste
- 24 almonds, unsalted
- 2 cups vanilla flavored coconut milk or more if required, unsweetened

Method:

1. Add all the ingredients in a blender and blend until smooth.
2. Pour into glasses and serve.

5. Green glow Smoothie

Serves: 2

Ingredients:

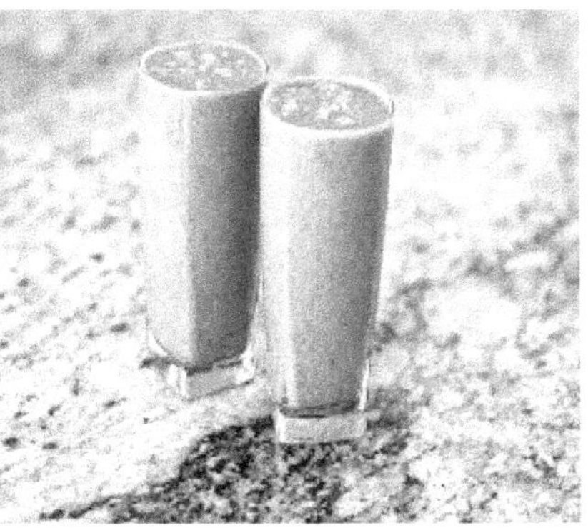

- 2 oranges, separated into segments, deseeded
- 4 cups dandelion greens or kale
- 2 medium ripe bananas, chopped
- 1 lime, peeled, chopped
- 2 inch piece ginger, peeled, sliced
- 2 tbsp chia seeds, soaked for about 5 minutes in water
- 2 cups almond milk or water

Method:

1. Add all the ingredients except dandelion greens to your blender. Blend until smooth.
2. Add the greens and blend until smooth.
3. Pour into glasses and serve with crushed ice.

6. **Healthy Chia and Oats Smoothie**

Serves: 2

Ingredients:

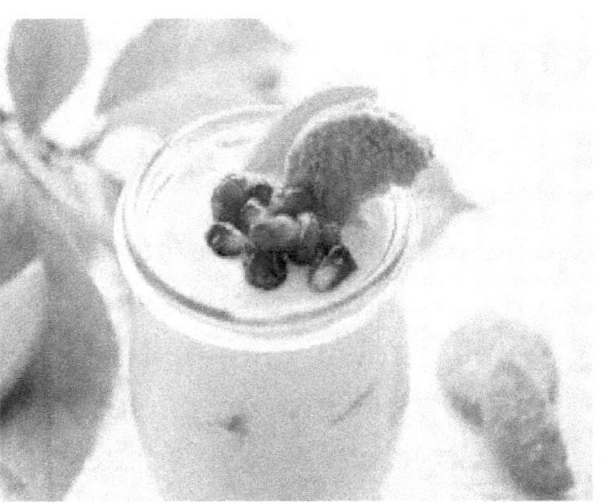

- 6 tbsp oats
- 2 tbsp chia seeds
- 2 tbsp hemp powder
- 4 medjool dates, pitted (optional)
- 2 bananas, chopped
- 1 cup almond milk
- 1 cup frozen berries
- 2 big handful's spinach, torn

Method:

1. Add all the ingredients in a blender and blend until smooth.
2. Pour in glasses and serve.

7. Cherry Almond and Cereal Smoothie

Serves: 2

Ingredients:

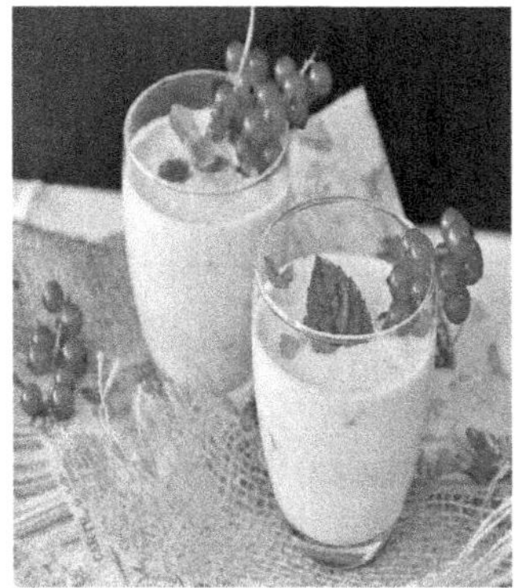

- 1 cup fresh cherries, pitted + extra to garnish
- ¼ cup rolled oats
- 1 tbsp hemp seeds
- 1 cup almond milk

Method:

1. Add all the ingredients in a blender and blend until smooth.
2. Pour into glasses and serve garnished with cherries.

8. Banana Orange Smoothie

Serves: 2

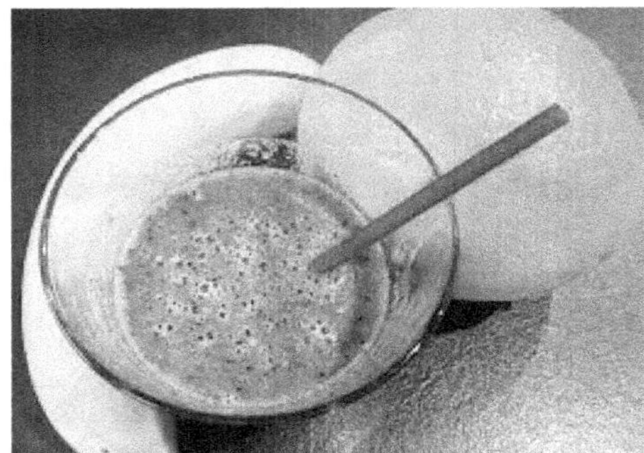

Ingredients:

- 2 cups fat free milk
- 1 cup nonfat Greek yogurt
- 1 medium banana
- 1 cup collard greens
- 1 orange, peeled, deseeded, separated into segments
- 6 strawberries, chopped
- 2 tbsp sesame seeds

Method:

1. Add all the ingredients in a blender and blend until smooth.
2. Pour in glasses and serve.

9. Crunchy Banana Yoghurt

Serves: 2

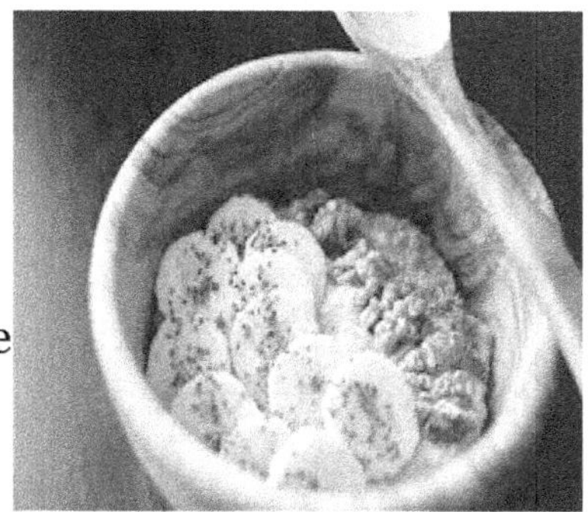

Ingredients:

- 3 cups fat free natural Greek style yogurt
- 1 ounce mixed seeds or nuts of your choice like pumpkin seeds etc.
- 2 bananas, sliced

Method:

1. Take 4 bowls and add ¾ cup yogurt into each bowl.
2. Divide the banana slices among the bowl.
3. Sprinkle seeds on top and serve.

10.   Grapefruit Yogurt Parfait

Serves: 4

Ingredients:

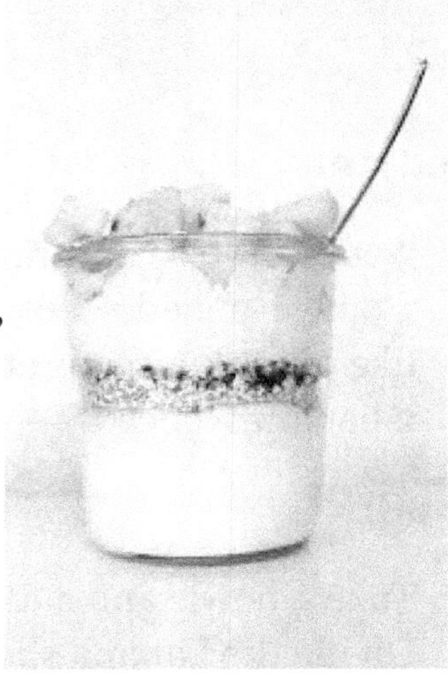

- ½ cup amaranth
- 1 grapefruit, peeled, separated into segments, deseeded, chopped
- 3 tbsp toasted coconut
- Stevia to taste (optional)
- 1 cup plain, nonfat yogurt
- 3 tbsp toasted coconut

Method:

1. Place a pan over medium heat. Add amaranth and let it pop. It should take 3-5 minutes. Let it cool for a few minutes.
2. Add yogurt into a bowl. Add stevia and stir. Add 2 tbsp yogurt into each of 4 glasses.
3. Place a layer of grapefruit in each glass. Add 1 tbsp popped amaranth and sprinkle some coconut into the glasses.
4. Repeat steps 2-3 until all the ingredients are used up.

11.   Creamy Mango and Banana Overnight Oats

Serves: 1

Ingredients:

For the smoothie:

- 1 ripe banana
- ½ mango, peeled, cubed
- ½ tbsp ground flaxseed
- 1 cup almond milk

For the oats:

- 1/3 cup oats
- 1 small ripe banana, mashed
- 1/2 cup almond milk
- ½ tbsp ground flaxseed
- 2 tbsp chia seeds
- Stevia or erythritol to taste

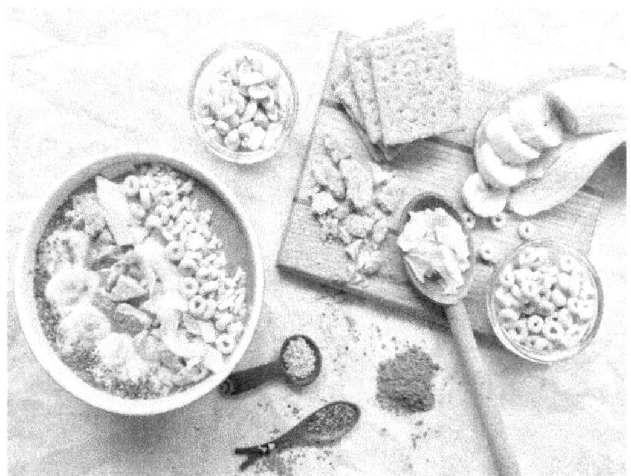

Method:

1. Add all the smoothie ingredients into a blender and blend until smooth.
2. Pour into a tall glass.
3. To make the oats layer: Add oats, almond milk, flaxseed, chia seeds and stevia into a bowl. Stir well and add banana. Mix until well combined. Pour it over the smoothie in the glass.
4. Chill in the refrigerator overnight and serve.

12.   Bacon and Eggs with Tomatoes

Serves: 4

Ingredients:

- 4 large ripe tomatoes, halved
- 8 rashers smoked back bacon, trimmed of fat
- 4 eggs
- Salt to taste
- Pepper to taste
- 1 tsp vinegar

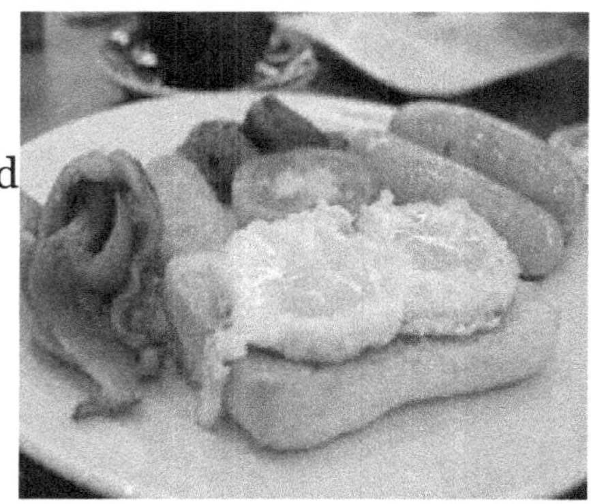

Method:

1. Set up the grill to preheat. Let it preheat to high heat.
2. Place a rack on the grill pan. Line the pan with foil. Place tomatoes on the rack. Let it grill for 3 minutes. Place bacon along with the tomatoes.
3. Grill for 4 minutes until soft.
4. Meanwhile, place a large saucepan over medium high heat. Fill the saucepan up to about ¾ with water. Let it boil.
5. When it begins to boil, add vinegar and stir. Crack an egg into a bowl and slowly slide the egg into the boiling water. Repeat this, one at a time.
6. Cook each egg until it is soft boiled, for 2-3 minutes.
7. Meanwhile, divide the bacon and tomatoes into 2 plates.
8. Remove the eggs with a slotted spoon and place on the plates. Sprinkle salt and pepper and serve.

13.   Cinnamon Porridge

Serves: 4

Ingredients:

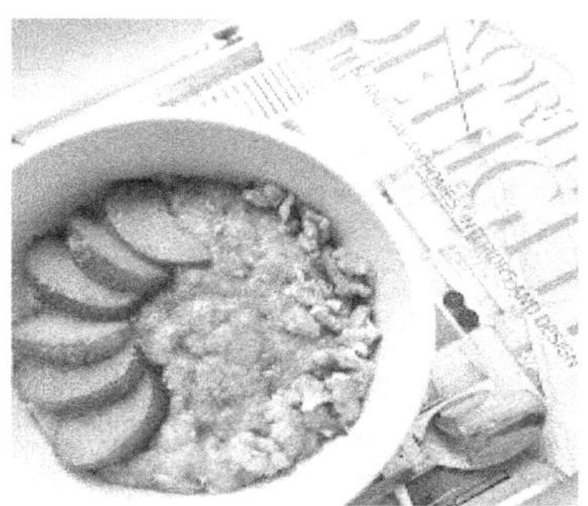

- 4 ½ ounces jumbo porridge oats
- 20 ounces semi-skimmed milk
- 1 tsp lemon juice
- ½ tsp ground cinnamon + extra to garnish
- 2 ripe medium pears, peeled, cored, grated

Method:

1. Add oats, milk and cinnamon into a nonstick saucepan. Place the saucepan over medium low heat. Cook until creamy. Stir constantly.
2. Divide into bowls. Scatter pear on top. Drizzle lemon juice on top. Garnish with cinnamon and serve.

14.   Spinach Omelet

Serves: 2

Ingredients:

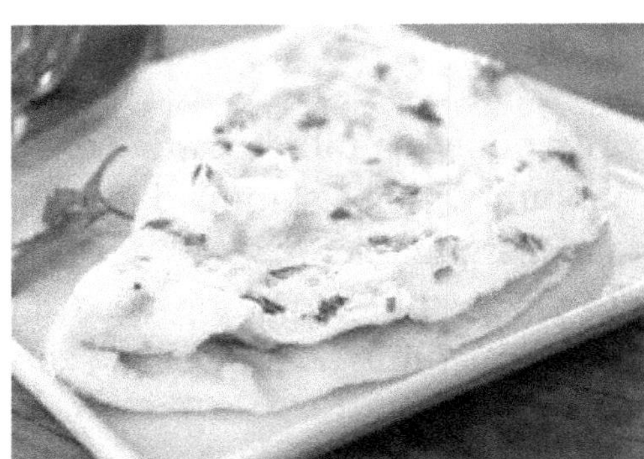

- 2 yolks
- 10 egg whites
- 1 tomato, chopped
- 2 tbsp chopped purple onion
- 2 handfuls spinach, shredded
- A handful basil, chopped
- 2 cloves garlic, minced (optional)
- 2 ounces almond milk
- Olive oil cooking spray

Method:

1. Whisk together yolks, whites and almond milk in a bowl.
2. Take a nonstick pan and place it over medium heat. Spray with cooking spray. When oil is heated, add onion, tomato and spinach and sauté for a couple of minutes.
3. Remove the vegetables and set aside.
4. Spray the pan with cooking spray. Let the pan heat.
5. Lower the heat and pour half the egg mixture into the pan. When the eggs are set, place half the vegetable mixture on one half of the omelet. Fold the other half over the filling.
6. Remove on to a serving plate and serve.
7. Repeat the steps 4-6 to make the other omelet.

15. Baked Moroccan Eggs

Serves: 4

Ingredients:

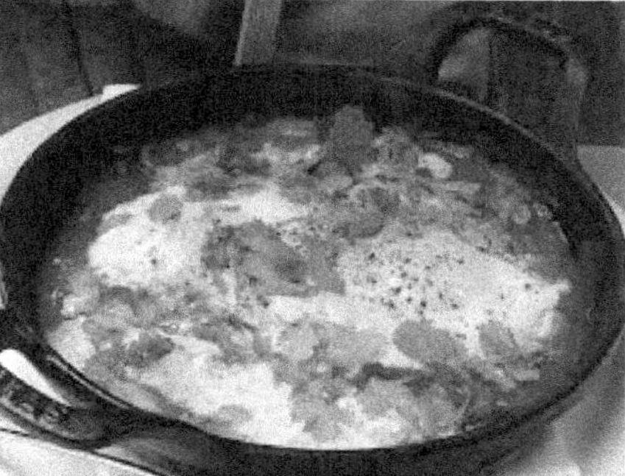

- 1 tbsp olive oil
- 2 cloves garlic, peeled, grated
- 28 ounces cherry tomatoes or grape tomatoes, chopped
- Freshly ground pepper powder
- 2 tbsp fresh cilantro or parsley, chopped
- 1 onion, chopped
- ½ tsp ground cinnamon
- 1 tsp ground coriander
- ½ tsp salt or to taste
- 1 tsp ras-el-hanout
- 4 large eggs

Method:

1. Place a pan over medium heat. Add oil. When the oil is heated, add onion and garlic and sauté until translucent.
2. Stir in the tomatoes, pepper powder and salt. Cook for 10-12 minutes.
3. Add water if you desire a sauce of thinner consistency. Add ras-el-hanout, ground coriander and cinnamon and mix well.
4. Transfer into 4 small ovenproof dishes. Crack an egg into each dish.
5. Bake in a preheated oven at 300 ° F for 12-15 minutes or until the eggs are cooked as per your liking.

16.　　Scrambled Eggs

Serves: 4

Ingredients:

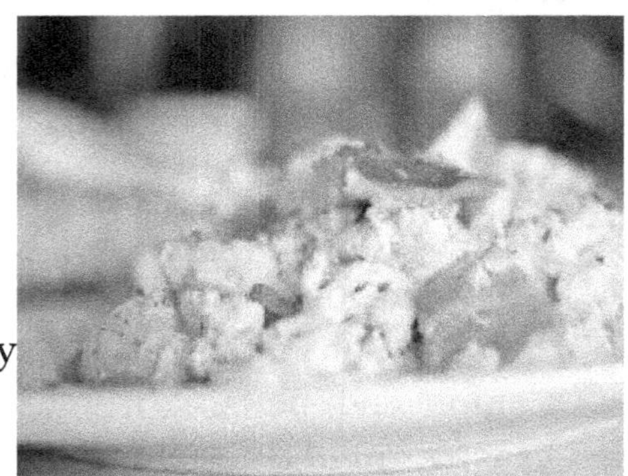

- 16 midi vine tomatoes, halved
- 6 large free range eggs
- 2 tbsp chopped chives
- Freshly ground black pepper to taste
- Low calorie cooking spray
- 2 ½ ounces smoked salmon, roughly chopped
- 2 ounces fresh watercress, to serve

Method:

1. Sprinkle pepper over the tomatoes.
2. Place a pan over medium heat. Spray with cooking spray.
3. When the pan heats, add tomatoes and sauté until soft. Stir occasionally. The tomatoes should not be broken down. Remove the tomatoes and place in a bowl.
4. Add eggs and pepper into a bowl and whisk well.
5. Add salmon and chives and stir.
6. Pour into the pan. Stir occasionally and cook until the eggs are scrambled and soft cooked. Turn off the heat and stir for 30-40 seconds.
7. Divide the tomatoes into 4 serving plates. Place scrambled eggs and watercress and serve.

17.   Garlic Mushroom Frittata

Serves: 4

Ingredients:

- 18 ounces chestnut mushrooms, sliced
- 2 tbsp thinly sliced fresh chives
- Freshly ground pepper to taste
- Low calorie cooking spray
- 2 small cloves garlic, crushed
- 8 large free range eggs, beaten

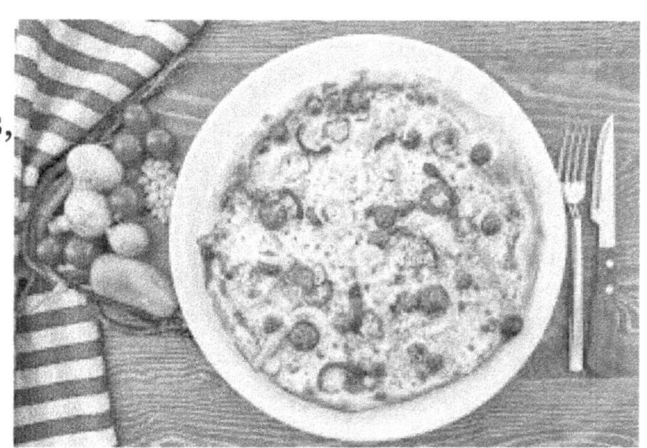

<u>For salad:</u>

- 2 little gem lettuce, leaves separated
- 2/3 cucumber, chopped
- 7 ounces cherry tomatoes, halved

Method:

1. Place a medium size heatproof pan over high heat. Spray with cooking spray. Add mushrooms and sauté for 2-3 minutes. Do not crowd and cook it in batches. Spray with oil each time. Remove the mushrooms and place in a strainer until all the mushrooms are cooked.
2. When all the mushrooms are cooked, add it back into the pan. Add garlic and chives and pepper and sauté for a minute. Lower the heat to low heat. Spread the mushrooms evenly in the pan.
3. Pour eggs into the pan. Do not stir. Cook for a few minutes until nearly set.
4. Transfer the pan into a preheated grill or broiler and grill until set.
5. Meanwhile, add all the salad ingredients into a bowl and toss well.
6. Run a knife around the edges of the frittata and invert on to a plate. Cut into wedges.
7. Serve with salad.

18.   Amaranth Pancakes

Serves: 8

Ingredients:

For dry ingredients:

- 1 ½ cups whole wheat flour
- 1 cup amaranth flour
- 1 tsp baking powder
- 1 tsp salt
- ½ tsp baking soda

For wet ingredients:

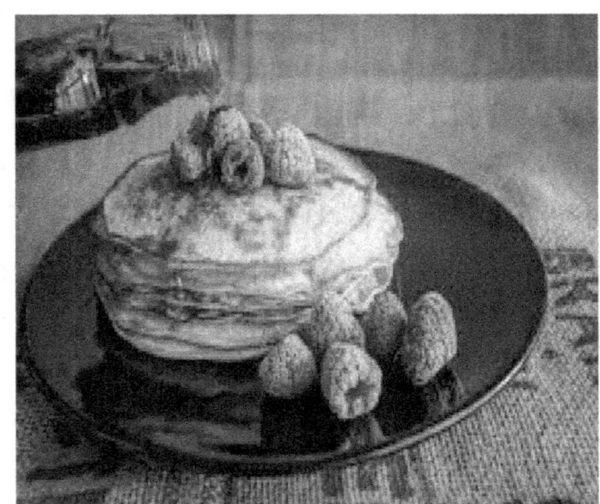

- 1 cup skim milk
- 2 cups buttermilk
- 6 tbsp butter, melted
- 2 eggs, beaten

Method:

1. Add all the dry ingredients into a bowl and stir.
2. Whisk together all the wet ingredients into another bowl. Pour into the bowl of dry ingredients and whisk until well combined.
3. Place a nonstick pan over medium heat. Pour 4-5 tbsp of batter on it. Swirl the pan so that the batter spreads.
4. Lower heat and cover with a lid. Bubbles will begin to appear on the pancake. Cook until the underside is golden brown. Flip sides and cook the other side too.
5. Repeat the previous step to make remaining pancakes.

19.   Five Grain Porridge

Serves: 4

Ingredients:

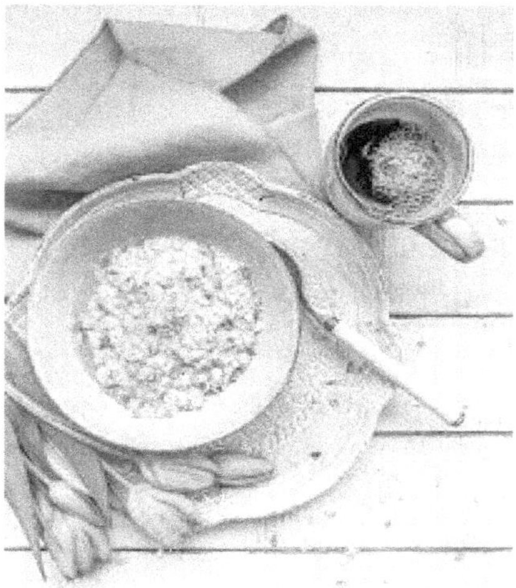

- ¼ cup brown rice
- 2 tbsp amaranth
- ¼ cup wheat bran
- ¼ cup quinoa
- 2 tbsp millet
- 3-4 cups water
- 1 apple, cored, sliced
- Stevia to taste
- ½ tsp ground cinnamon
- 2 tbsp coconut flakes
- Sea salt to taste
- Bee pollen to sprinkle

Method:

1. Add all the grains into a bowl. Rinse and add into a saucepan. Add water and stir. Place saucepan over medium heat. When it begins to boil, lower the heat and simmer until cooked. Add stevia and stir.
2. Meanwhile, place a nonstick pan over medium heat. Place apple slices and sprinkle cinnamon over it. Cook until apples are brown.
3. Serve porridge in bowls. Place apple slices on top. Sprinkle coconut flakes and bee pollen on top and serve.

20.   Quinoa Veggie Porridge

Serves: 4

Ingredients:

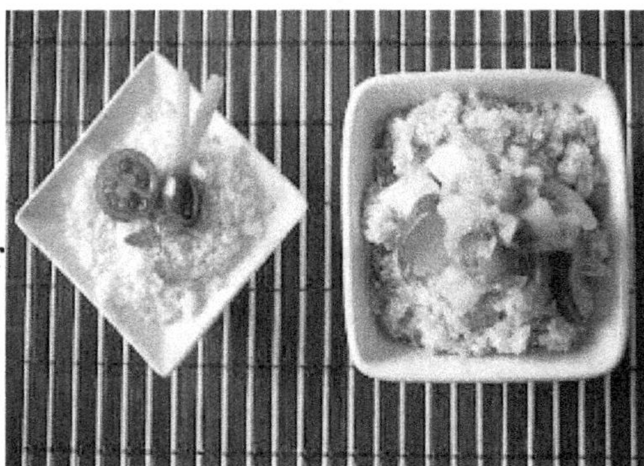

- 1 onion, chopped
- ½ cup kuri squash or any other squash, chopped
- 1 small piece kombu sea vegetable
- 1 stalk celery, chopped
- ¼ cup quinoa, rinsed
- 2 green onions, thinly sliced, on the diagonal
- 4 cups water
- Miso to taste

Method:

1. Add all the ingredients except miso into a heavy bottom saucepan. Cover and cook until tender. Stir frequently.
2. Add miso and little of the liquid from the porridge. Stir and add into the porridge. Stir and serve.

21. Multigrain Porridge

Serves: 8

Ingredients:

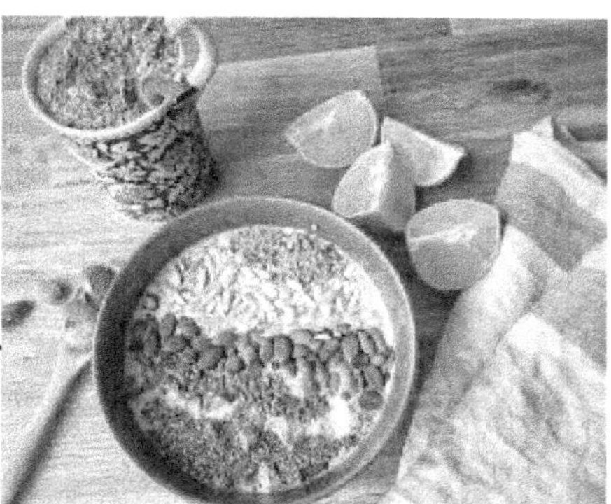

- 2 tbsp each of bulgur, oats, quinoa, millet, and buckwheat, soaked in water overnight, drained
- 6 cups water
- 2 cups almond milk or any other milk of your choice
- Sweetener to taste like stevia or swerve (optional)

Method:

1. Add all the grains and water into a heavy bottom saucepan. Place saucepan over high heat. When it begins to boil, lower the heat and cover with a lid. Simmer until the grains are cooked. Stir frequently.
2. Add sweetener and milk and serve.

22. Buckwheat Porridge

Serves: 2

Ingredients:

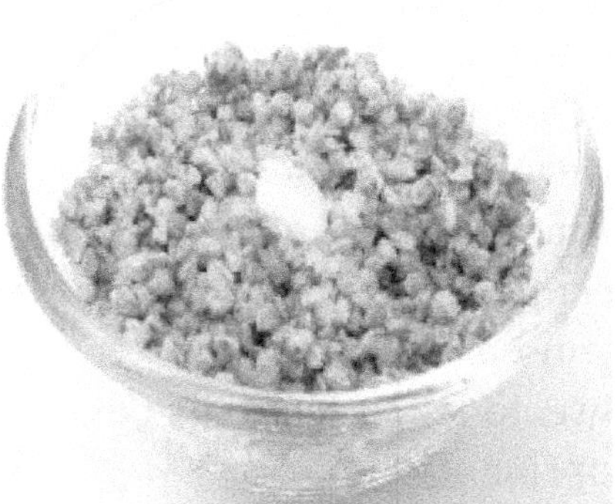

- ½ cup buckwheat groats, rinsed
- 1 small banana, sliced
- 1 ½ cups rice milk + extra to serve
- 2 tbsp raisins
- ¼ cup mixed nuts (almonds and walnuts)
- ¼ tsp vanilla
- ½ tsp ground cinnamon

Method:

1. Add all the ingredients except the nuts into a heavy bottom saucepan. Place saucepan over high heat. When it begins to boil, lower the heat and simmer until the groats are cooked. Stir frequently.
2. Ladle into bowls.
3. Add nuts and milk and serve.

23.   Savory Wheat Porridge

Serves: 3

Ingredients:

- 3 1/2 ounces wheat, rinsed, drained
- 3 1/2 ounces meat, boneless, cut into small cubes
- 3 cups water
- 1 small stick cinnamon
- 2 cloves garlic, chopped
- 1 tsp Maggi CukupRasa
- 1 medium carrot, diced, blanched
- 1 tbsp corn oil
- ½ tsp cumin powder
- ½ tsp aniseed powder
- ½ red chili, thinly sliced
- 2 ½ tbsp water
- 1 small cucumber, cut into matchsticks
- Salt to taste

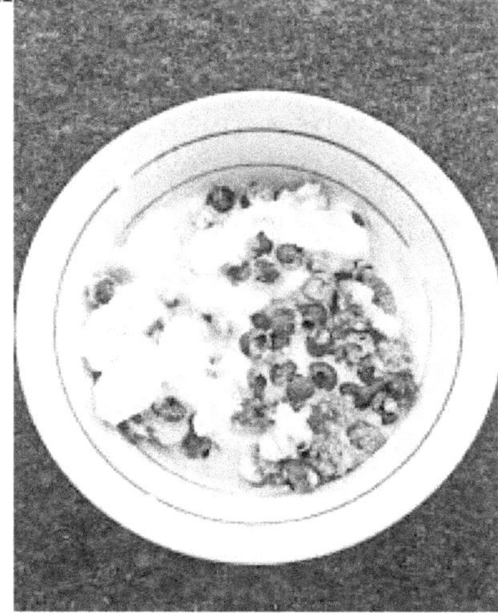

Method:

1. Add 3 cups water, meat, cinnamon and wheat into a pot. Bring to a boil.
2. Lower the heat and simmer until tender. Stir occasionally.
3. Meanwhile, place a pan over medium heat. Add corn oil. When the oil is heated, add garlic, carrot, cumin, coriander and aniseed powders and 2-½ tbsp water. Sauté until the oil begins to shine around the edges of the pan. Turn off the heat.
4. When the wheat is tender, add the carrot mixture into the pot. Stir and simmer for 5 minutes. Add salt to taste.
5. Ladle into bowls. Top with cucumber and chili and salt.

24. Brown Rice, Lentils and Green Tea Porridge

Serves: 8

Ingredients:

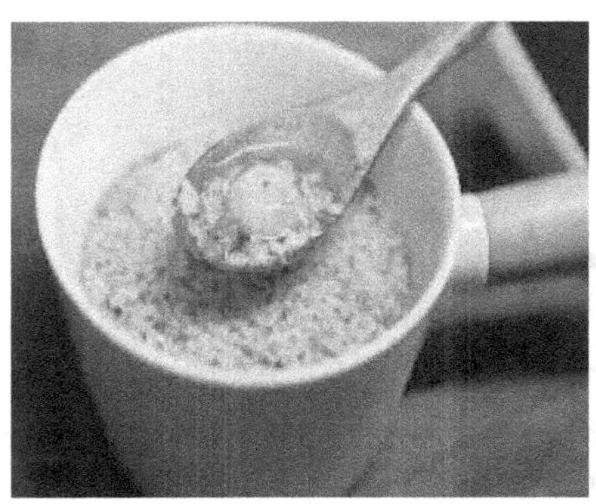

- 2 cups short grain brown rice, rinsed
- 6 green tea bags
- ½ cup brown lentils, rinsed
- 12 cups water
- Salt to taste

<u>To serve:</u> (optional, use any or all of them)

- Sesame seeds, salted, toasted
- Tamari sauce to taste
- Miso to taste
- Umiboshi plum pickle

Method:

1. Add all the ingredients into a Dutch oven. Cover with the lid.
2. Discard tea bags.
3. Ladle into bowls. Serve with any of the optional toppings.

25. Barbeque Pork Ribs

Serves: 3-4

Ingredients:

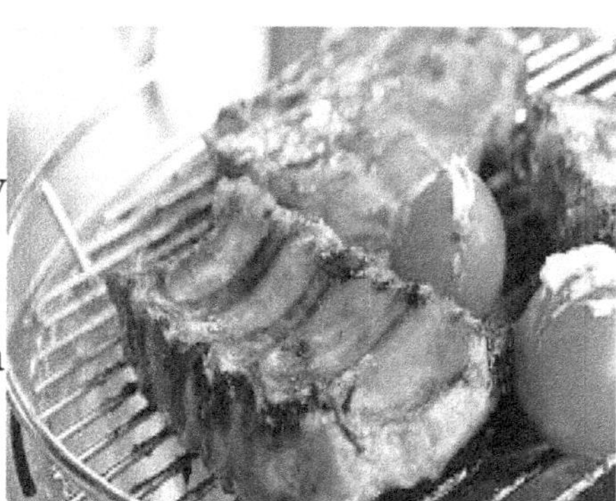

- 2-2 ½ pounds pork spareribs or baby back ribs
- 1 tsp liquid smoke (optional)
- ½ cup low carb barbecue sauce + extra to serve
- 2 tbsp Dijon mustard
- ½ cup spice rub

Method:

1. Place a sheet of aluminum foil on a rimmed baking sheet. Place a wire rack over it.
2. Place the ribs on the rack with the meat side facing up. Do not overlap.
3. Add mustard and liquid smoke into a bowl and stir. Brush this mixture all over the ribs.
4. Sprinkle dry rub over the ribs and press lightly so that the rub sticks on to the ribs.
5. Place in a preheated oven with broiler setting. Broil until the ribs are brown.
6. Place a rack in the center of the oven. Shift the ribs onto this rack.
7. Bake in a preheated oven at 300 ° F for 2-3 hours if using spareribs or for 1 ½ -2 hours if using baby back ribs.
8. Cover the ribs with foil when the meat is half cooked.

9. Baste with barbecue sauce during the last 30 minutes of cooking. Cover and continue baking.
10. To check if the meat is cooked, insert a knife in the thickest part of the meat. If it pierces easily, the meat is cooked else cook it for some more time.
11. When done, let the meat sit for 10 minutes. Do not remove the foil during this time.
12. Uncover and place on your cutting board. When cool enough to handle, separate the ribs by cutting in between the bones.
13. Serve with extra barbecue sauce.

26.   Roast Pork with Apples & Onions

Serves: 3

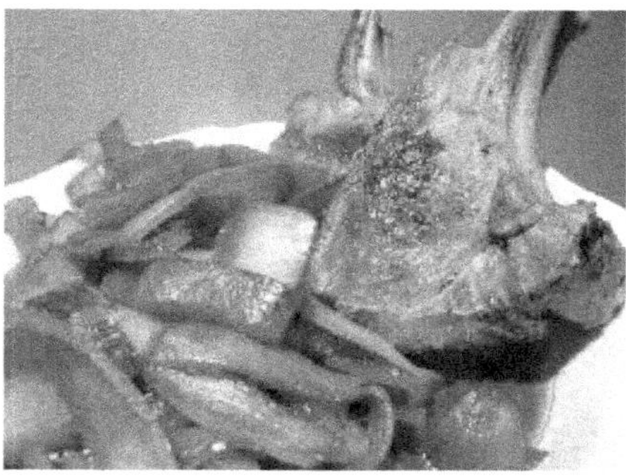

Ingredients:

- 1 pound pork loin roast
- Salt to taste
- Pepper to taste
- ½ tbsp olive oil
- 1 large onion, cut into ¾ inch wedges
- ½ tbsp minced fresh rosemary or ½ tsp dried rosemary, crushed
- 2 Golden Delicious apples, cut into 1 inch wedges
- 3 cloves garlic, peeled
- Low calorie cooking spray

Method:

1. Spray a roasting pan with cooking spray.
2. Season roast with salt and pepper. Place a nonstick skillet over medium heat. Add oil. When the oil is heated, add roast and cook until brown all over. Transfer into the prepared roasting pan. Lay the apple, garlic and onion slices all around the roast. Scatter rosemary.
3. Roast for 40-45 minutes or until an instant read thermometer shows 145° F when inserted in the thickest part of the meat.
4. Remove meat and cover with foil. Let it rest for 10 minutes.
5. Slice roast and serve with apple, garlic and onions.

27.Mediterranean Pork and Orzo

Serves: 3

Ingredients:

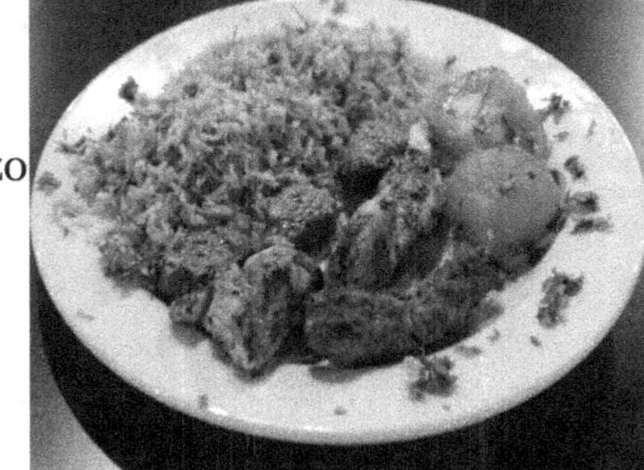

- ¾ pound pork tenderloin
- 1 tbsp olive oil
- 2/3 cup uncooked whole wheat orzo pasta
- 3 ounces fresh baby spinach
- 6 tbsp reduced fat feta cheese
- ½ tsp coarsely ground pepper
- 1 ½ quarts water
- ¼ tsp salt or to taste
- ½ cup grape tomatoes, halved

Method:

1. Season pork with pepper. Rub it well into it. Chop into 1-inch chunks.
2. Place a nonstick skillet over medium heat. Add oil. When the oil is heated, add pork and sauté until it is not pink anymore.
3. Meanwhile, place a pot of water over high heat. When it begins to boil, add orzo and salt and simmer for 8-9 minutes or until al dente. Add spinach and turn off the heat after a minute. Drain.
4. Add orzo into the skillet. Also add tomatoes, pork and feta and toss well. Heat thoroughly and serve.

28.   Southwestern Pineapple Pork Chops

Serves: 8

Ingredients:

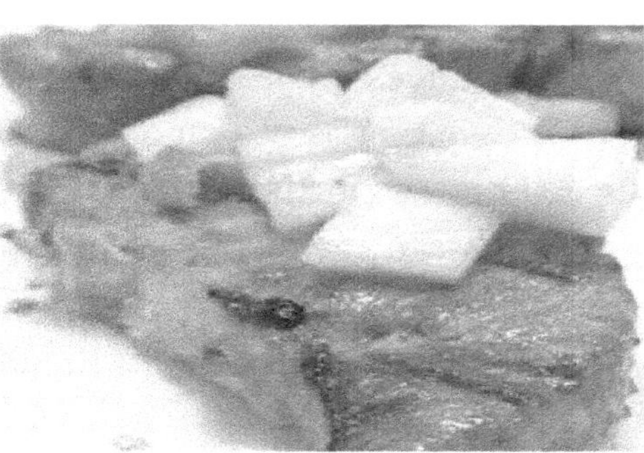

- 8 pork loin chops (5 ounces each), boneless
- 2 tbsp canola oil
- 2 cups medium salsa
- 1 tsp garlic pepper blend
- 2 cans (8 ounces each) unsweetened crushed pineapple with its liquid
- A handful fresh cilantro, minced

Method:

1. Season pork with pepper.
2. Place a nonstick skillet over medium heat. Add oil. When the oil is heated, add pork and sauté until brown. Remove with a slotted spoon and set aside.
3. Add pineapple and salsa into the skillet and stir. When it begins to boil, add pork and stir until well coated.
4. Lower the heat and cover with a lid. Cook until tender.
5. Garnish with cilantro and serve.

29. Stir-fried Pork with Ginger and Soy Sauce

Serves: 4

Ingredients:

- 18 ounces pork tenderloin, trimmed of fat, chopped into chunks
- 4 tbsp dark soy sauce
- 11 ounces button mushrooms, sliced
- 5 ounces mange tout, trimmed
- 2 cloves garlic, thinly sliced
- Freshly ground pepper to taste
- 2 tsp cornflour mixed with 4 tbsp cold water
- Low calorie cooking spray
- 4 red peppers, deseeded, sliced
- 1 ounce fresh ginger, peeled, cut into matchsticks
- 8 spring onions, cut into 2 inch pieces

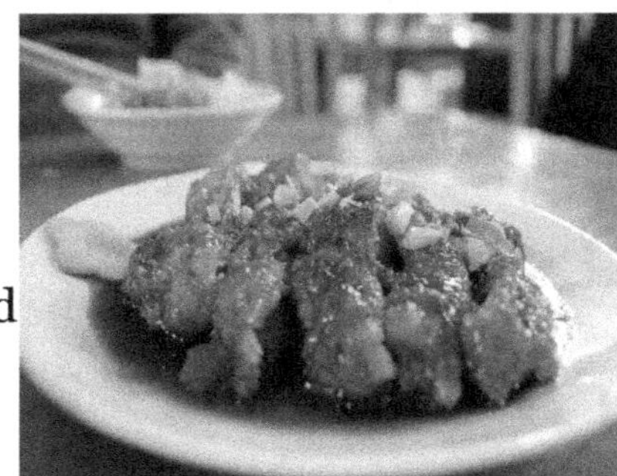

Method:

1. Sprinkle pepper over the pork. Add corn flour mixture and soy sauce into a bowl and stir.
2. Place a large wok over high heat. Spray with cooking spray. Add pork and sauté for a couple of minutes until light brown but it should not be fully cooked.
3. Remove with a slotted spoon and set aside on a plate.
4. Spray more oil in the wok. Lower the heat to medium heat.
5. Add ginger, mushrooms and pepper and cook for 2-3 minutes. Stir in the mange tout and cook for a minute.
6. Stir in the garlic, ginger and spring onions and cook for a few seconds until fragrant.
7. Add pork and mix well. Stir in the cornflour mixture. Stir constantly until thick.
8. Serve.

30. Chorizo Spaghetti Squash Pasta

Serves: 6

Ingredients:

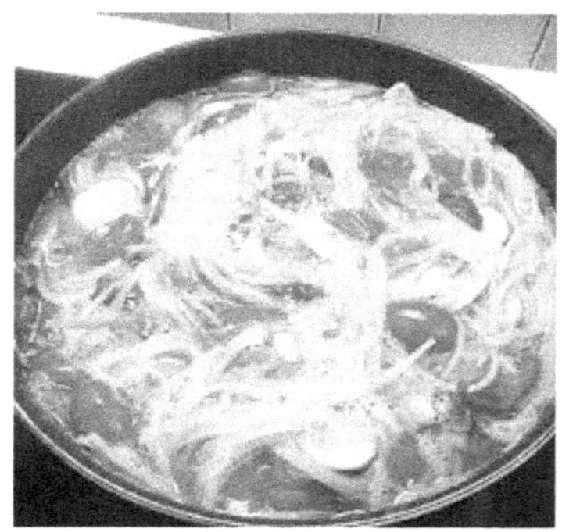

- 2 large spaghetti squashes, halved crosswise
- 2 cups kale or spinach (optional)
- 2 cans (28 ounces each) crushed tomatoes
- A handful fresh basil, to garnish
- 2 pounds chorizo
- 1 1/3 pounds chicken broth
- Salt to taste

Method:

1. Place a sheet of parchment paper over a large baking sheet. Place the squash on it, with the cut side facing down.
2. Bake in a preheated oven at 425 ° F for 35-45 minutes or until tender. When done, turn the squash so that it cools. When cool enough to handle, using a fork, pull strands of spaghetti squash and set aside.
3. Place a Dutch oven over medium heat. Add chorizo and cook until brown. Break it simultaneously as it cooks.
4. Add spinach and cook until it wilts. Add broth and tomatoes and mix well. Stir in the spaghetti squash. Mix until well combined.
5. Lower the heat and simmer for 8-10 minutes. Add salt and stir.
6. Garnish with basil and serve.

31. Pig Rib Salad

Serves: 2

Ingredients:

- 1 rack leftover cooked pork ribs, remove meat from the bones, chopped
- 3-4 tsp Sriracha sauce
- 1 cucumber, sliced
- 1 large carrot, peeled, shredded
- 1 small red onion, thinly sliced
- 4-6 tbsp homemade dressing of your choice
- 5-6 cups romaine lettuce, shredded

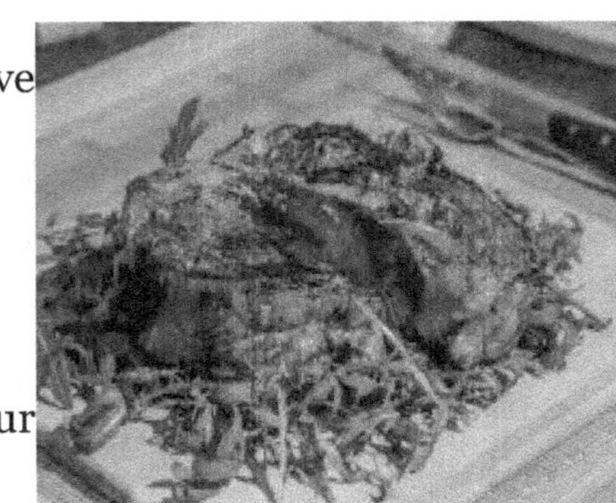

Method:

1. Add all the ingredients into a bowl. Toss well and serve.

32. Steak with Hawaiian Rice

Serves: 2

Ingredients:

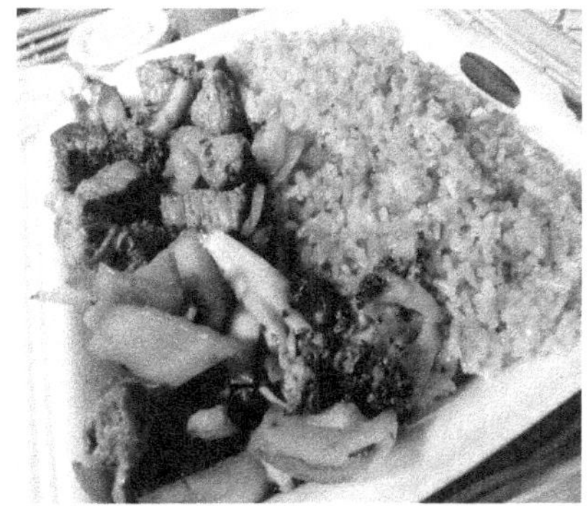

- ¾ pound cooked skirt steak, thinly sliced
- 1 cup fresh pineapple chunks
- 1 ½ cups cooked rice
- 1 tsp chili powder
- ¼ tsp salt
- Lime wedges to serve

Method:

1. Place a nonstick skillet over medium heat. Add rice and pineapple and stir-fry for 3-4 minutes. Sprinkle salt and chili powder and stir. Add cilantro and stir.
2. Divide rice into plates. Place steak on top and serve with lime wedges.

33. Beef and Portobello Bourguignon

Serves: 8

Ingredients:

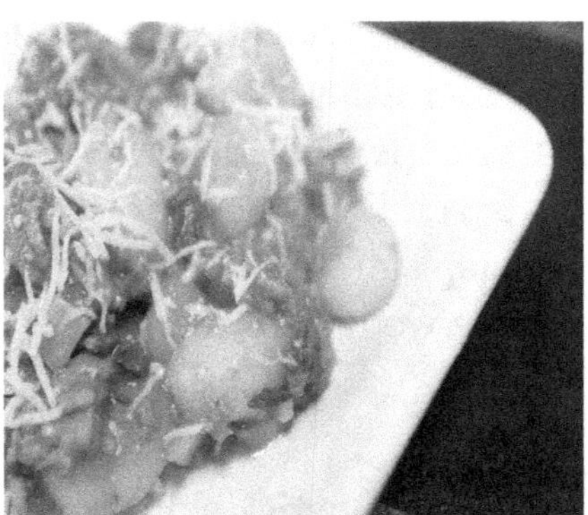

- 4 slices bacon
- Salt to taste
- Pepper to taste
- 1 ½ tbsp cornstarch
- 2 cups water
- 60 ounces Portobello mushroom caps
- 2 pounds beef chuck
- 2 large onions, chopped
- 4 cups dry red wine
- 4 cloves garlic, sliced
- 2 pounds carrots, chopped into chunks
- A handful fresh rosemary leaves, minced

Method:

1. Place a large, heavy stockpot or Dutch oven over medium high heat.
2. Add bacon and cook until crisp. Remove with a slotted spoon and place on a plate lined with paper towels.
3. Sprinkle beef with salt and pepper and place in the pot, in a single layer. Cook until brown all over. Remove with a slotted spoon and place in a bowl.
4. Add onion and garlic into the pot and sauté until translucent. Add cornstarch and stir constantly for a minute.
5. Pour water and wine, stirring constantly. Keep stirring until it thickens.
6. Add carrots and beef along with the cooked juices. Turn off the heat. Fasten the lid and transfer the pot into an oven.
7. Bake in a preheated oven at 425 ° F for 60-75 minutes or until meat is cooked.

8. Add mushroom and rosemary and stir. Fasten the lid and continue baking for 30-35 minutes or until the mushroom is cooked.
9. Season with salt and pepper. Garnish with bacon and serve.

34.   Fried Egg Sandwich with BBQ Bacon

Serves: 2

Ingredients:

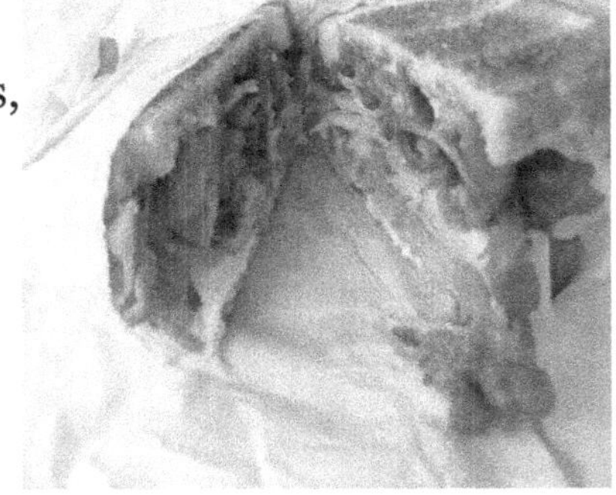

- 4 country-style whole wheat bread slices, ½ inch thick
- 2 low fat cheese slices
- 4 BBQ bacon slices
- 2 fried eggs
- 1-2 tbsp butter, melted
- 1 cup butter lettuce, chopped
- 2 tbsp mayonnaise

Method:

1. Place the oven rack 5 inches away from the heating element and set the oven for broiler setting.
2. Apply butter on the bread with a brush. Place on a baking sheet that is lined with foil.
3. Broil for a couple of minutes or until it is toasted lightly. Flip sides and broil for a couple of minutes.
4. Place a slice of cheese on each of 2 bread slices. Top with ½ cup lettuce and 2 bacon slices. Place a fried egg on top.
5. Apply mayonnaise on 2 slices of bread. Cover the sandwich with these 2 slices of bread, with the mayonnaise side facing down.
6. Serve.

35.Beefy Corn and Black Bean Chili

Serves: 2-3

Ingredients:

- ½ pound ground round
- ½ package (from a 14 ounces package) seasoned corn and black beans
- ½ can (from a 15 ounces can) seasoned tomato sauce for chili
- 1 green onion, sliced, to garnish (optional)
- Reduced fat sour cream, to garnish (optional)
- 1 tsp chili powder
- 1 cup beef broth

Method:

1. Place a Dutch oven over medium high heat. Add beef and chili powder and cook until brown. Break it simultaneously as it cooks. Drain the fat remaining in the pan.
2. Add corn mixture, tomato sauce and broth and stir.
3. When it begins to boil, lower the heat and cover with a lid. Simmer for 5-6 minutes. Remove the lid and simmer for another 3-4 minutes. Stir occasionally.
4. Divide into bowls. Garnish with sour cream and green onion and serve.

36. Salsa Meat Loaves

Serves: 8 (1 meatloaf per serving)

Ingredients:

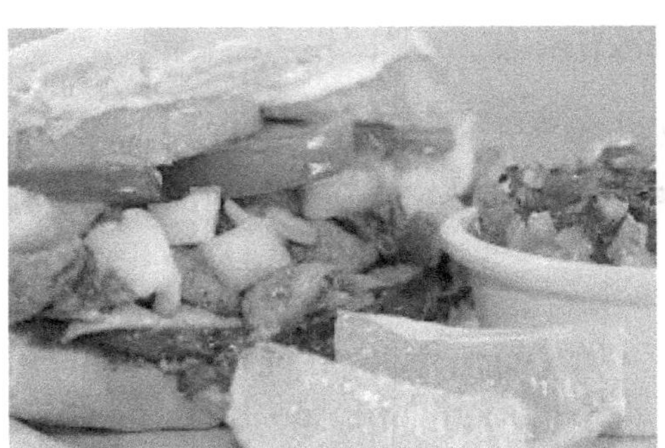

- 4 large egg white
- 1 ¼ cups chipotle salsa, divided
- 2 pounds extra lean ground beef
- 2/3 cup quick cooking oats
- ½ cup low carb ketchup, divided
- Low calorie cooking spray

Method:

1. Grease a large, rimmed baking sheet with cooking spray.
2. Add whites into a large mixing bowl and whisk well. Add oats, ¼ cup ketchup and 1-cup salsa and mix well.
3. Add beef and mix until well incorporated. Make 8 equal portions of the mixture. Shape into loaves of oval shape and place on the prepared baking sheet.
4. Bake in a preheated oven at 350 ° F for 30-45 minutes or until done.
5. Mix together in a bowl, remaining salsa and ketchup. Spread over the top of the loaves and serve.

37. Italian Style Meatballs with Courgette Pasta

Serves: 4

Ingredients:

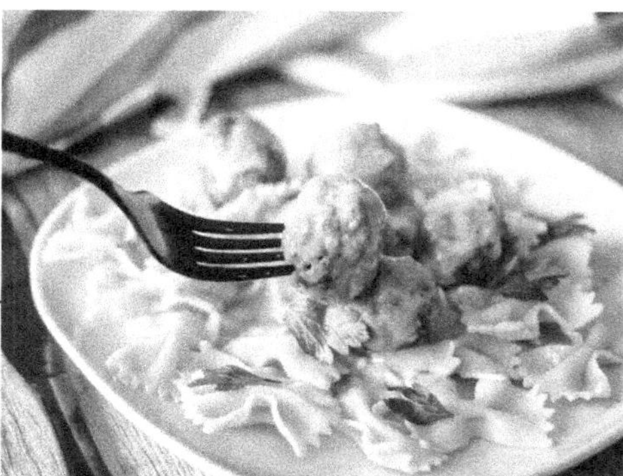

- 18 ounces extra lean beef mince (5% fat or lesser)
- 2 tsp dried mixed herbs
- 2 cloves garlic, crushed
- ¼ cup fresh basil leaves, finely shredded + extra to garnish
- 1 large onion, minced
- Low calorie cooking spray
- 2 cans (8 ounces each) chopped tomatoes
- Salt to taste
- Pepper to taste
- 4 medium courgettes, trimmed

Method:

1. Add beef, half the onions, salt, pepper and 1 tsp dried herbs into a mixing bowl. Mix until well combined.
2. Divide the mixture into 20 portions and shape into balls.
3. Place a nonstick pan over medium heat. Spray with cooking spray. Cook the meatballs in batches until brown all over. Remove the meatballs and set aside on a plate.
4. Add remaining onions into the pan and cook until translucent. Add garlic and sauté until fragrant.
5. Add tomatoes, herbs, basil and 2-½ cups water and stir frequently until it begins to boil.
6. Lower the heat and add meatballs. Cook for 20 minutes or until the meatballs are cooked.
7. Meanwhile, place a pot of water over high heat. Make ribbons of the courgette using a vegetable peeler. Drop the ribbons in the boiling water

for a minute. Drain and divide into 4 plates. Serve meatballs with sauce over it. Sprinkle basil on top and serve.

38.   Steak and Broccoli Stir Fry

Serves: 4

Ingredients:

- 8 ounces butter + extra to serve
- 18 ounces broccoli, chop the florets and stems
- 2 tbsp tamari sauce (optional)
- Salt to taste
- Pepper to taste
- 1 ½ pounds rib eye steaks, sliced
- 2 yellow onion, sliced
- 2 tbsp pumpkin seeds (pepitas)

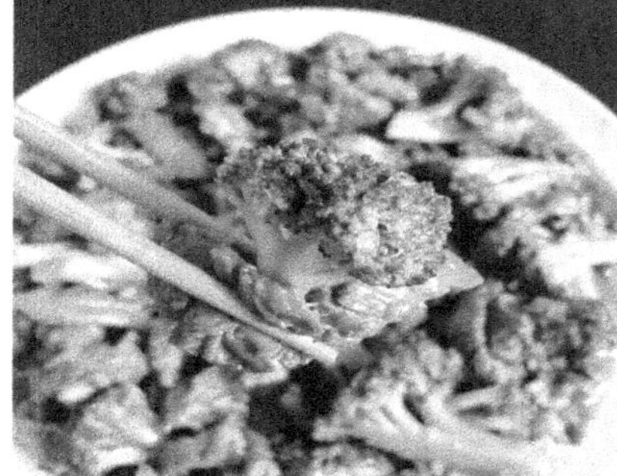

Method:

1. Place a wok or frying pan over medium heat. Add half the butter. When butter melts, place steak slices in the pan and cook until brown. Flip sides and cook the other side until brown. Sprinkle salt and pepper. Mix well.
2. Remove steaks with a slotted spoon and place on a plate.
3. Add remaining butter; add more if required.
4. Add broccoli and onions into the pan. Cook for 3-4 minutes or until tender.
5. Add tamari and mix well. Add steak back into the pan and stir. Taste and adjust the seasonings if necessary.
6. Serve right away with some butter and pumpkin seeds.

39. Skillet Steak with Potatoes and Herb Butter

Serves: 2

Ingredients:

- 1 lean New York strip steak
- ½ pound Yukon gold potatoes, cut into ½ inch thick slices
- ½ tbsp olive oil
- ½ tsp chopped thyme
- ½ tsp chopped oregano
- ½ tsp chopped rosemary
- ½ tbsp butter
- 2 cloves garlic, minced
- Salt to taste
- Pepper to taste

<u>For garlic herb butter:</u>

- 2 tbsp butter, softened
- ½ tsp chopped thyme
- ½ tsp chopped oregano
- ½ tsp chopped rosemary
- 2 cloves garlic, minced

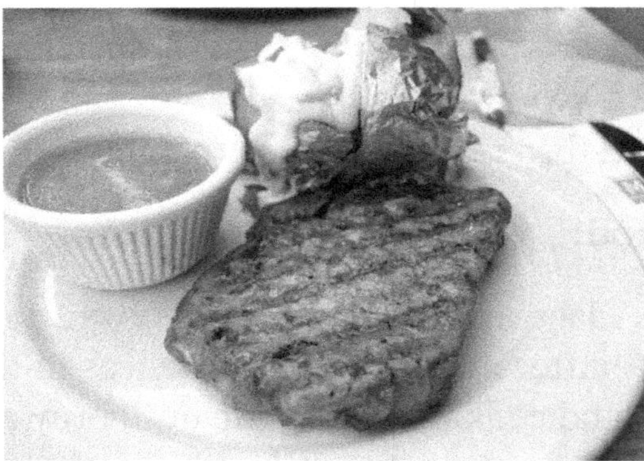

Method:

1. Place a skillet over medium high heat and allow it to heat. Add olive oil and butter. When butter melts, add potatoes, garlic and herbs. Cook for 3 minutes. Flip sides and cook for another 3 minutes or until tender. Remove potatoes and set aside on a plate.
2. Raise heat to high heat and place steak in the skillet. Cook until brown on both the sides.

3. Lower the heat to medium heat and cook until the way you like it cooked (rare, medium or well cooked).
4. Make the herb butter just before you remove steak from the pan.
5. Add all the ingredients of herb butter into a bowl and stir. Spread over the steak. Add potatoes into the pan and heat thoroughly.
6. Turn off the heat and serve.

40. Extra-Lean Burger and Salad

Serves: 4

Ingredients:

<u>For burger:</u>

- 1 small onion, finely chopped
- 18 ounces extra-lean beef mince (less than 5% fat)
- Freshly ground black pepper to taste
- 7 ounces Portobello mushrooms, finely chopped
- A handful fresh thyme, finely chopped or 1 tsp dried thyme
- Low calorie cooking spray

<u>For salad:</u>

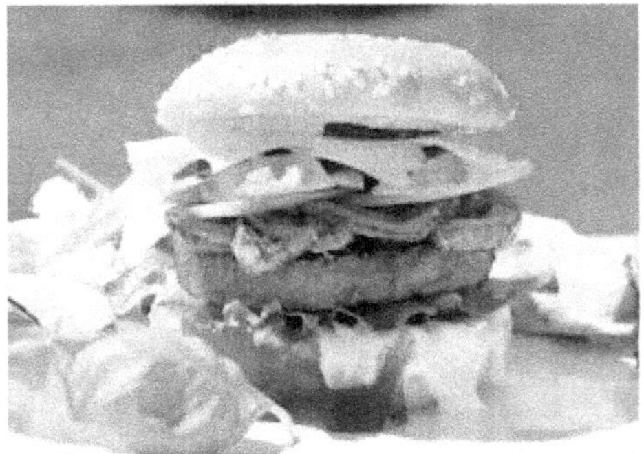

- 2 little gem lettuce, leaves separated
- 1 small cucumber, sliced
- 5 ounces cherry tomatoes, sliced

Method:

1. Place a pan over medium heat. Spray with cooking spray. Add onion and mushrooms and sauté for a few minutes until tender. Transfer into a bowl. Let it cool for 8-10 minutes.
2. Add beef, pepper and thyme and mix well using your hands. Divide the mixture into 4 equal portions and shape into burgers of about ¾ inch thickness.
3. Wipe the pan clean and place the pan back over medium low heat. Spray with cooking spray. Let the pan heat.
4. Place the burgers over it and cook until the underside is golden brown. Flip sides and cook the other side until golden brown and done inside.
5. Place lettuce leaves on serving plates. Place burgers over it. Top with tomato and cucumber slices and serve.

41. Cowboy Beef

Serves: 6

Ingredients:

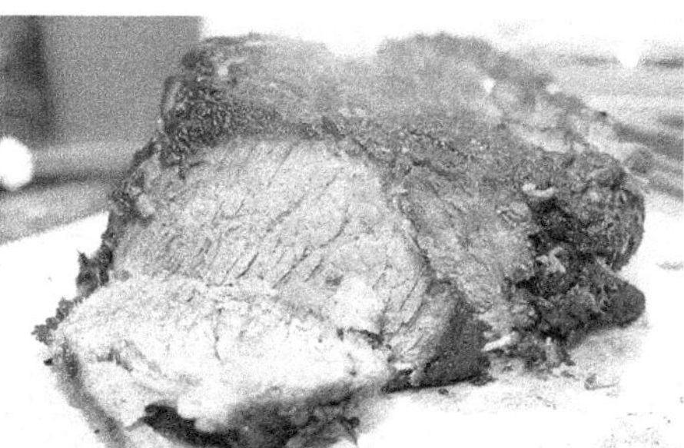

- 3 pounds beef chuck pot roast, boneless, trimmed of fat
- 1 ½ cans (11 ounces each) whole corn kernels with sweet peppers, drained
- 1 ½ cans (15 ounces each) chili beans in chili gravy
- 1 ½ cans (10 ounces each) diced tomatoes with green chilies with its liquid
- Salt to taste
- Pepper to taste
- 3 tsp canned, finely chopped chipotle pepper in adobo sauce
- Low calorie cooking spray

Method:

1. Spray the inside of a Dutch oven with cooking spray. Place the roast in it.
2. Mix together in a bowl, the rest of the ingredients and pour over the roast.
3. Cover and cook until meat is tender.
4. When done, remove meat and place on your cutting board. When cool enough to handle, slice and place in a serving dish. Pour rest of the ingredients over the meat and serve.

42. Cream of Chicken Soup

Serves: 4

Ingredients:

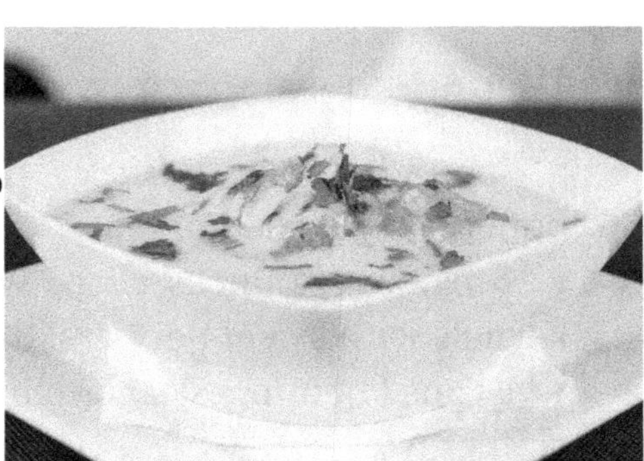

- 2 medium cauliflowers, broken into florets
- 2 cups chicken broth
- 1 tsp sea salt
- Freshly ground pepper to taste
- ¼ tsp dried thyme
- ½ cup chicken thighs, cooked, finely chopped
- 1 1/3 cups almond milk, unsweetened
- 2 tsp onion powder
- ½ tsp garlic powder
- ¼ tsp celery seeds (optional)
- ½ cup Collagen protein beef gelatin (optional)

Method:

1. Add all the ingredients except chicken and gelatin into a saucepan.
2. Place saucepan over medium heat. Cover with a lid.
3. When it begins to boil, lower heat. Simmer until cauliflower is soft.
4. Turn off the heat. Take out about a cup of the cooked liquid and add into a bowl.
5. Add gelatin, a tsp at a time into the bowl of cooked liquid. Whisk well each time until the gelatin is dissolved.
6. Pour the gelatin mixture into a blender. Also add the cooked cauliflower mixture.
7. Blend until smooth and creamy.
8. Pour the soup back into the pot. Place the pot over low heat.
9. Add chicken and stir. Cover and cook until the soup is heated thoroughly.

10. Ladle into soup bowls and serve.

43.Pan Fried Italian Chicken Thighs

Serves: 2

Ingredients:

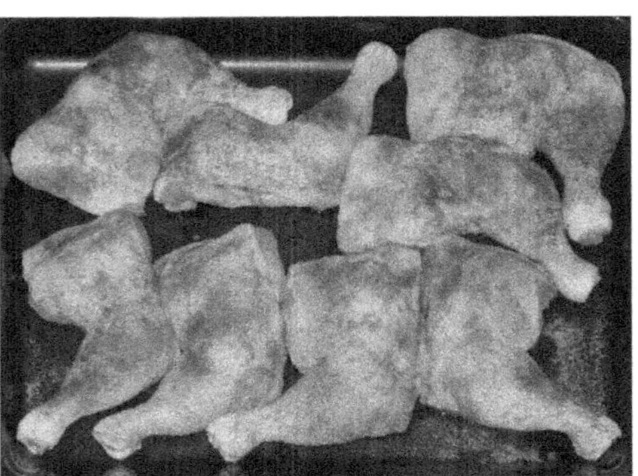

- 2 large chicken thighs
- ½ tbsp coconut oil or olive oil
- Freshly ground pepper to taste
- Kosher salt to taste
- Garlic powder to taste (optional)
- Paprika to taste (optional)
- ½ tsp Herbes de Provence
- ½ tsp dried basil
- ½ tsp dried oregano

Method:

1. Place a stainless steel or cast – iron skillet over medium heat. Add oil and let the pan heat.
2. Season the chicken on the skin side with some of the salt, pepper, herbs and spices if using.
3. Place chicken in the skillet, skin side down. Do not stir or move the chicken around. Sprinkle remaining herbs, spices, pepper and salt.
4. Cook for 20-25 minutes without covering. Cook until golden brown and the fat is released. If the skin sticks to the skillet, it means that it is not yet cooked on the skin side.
5. Flip sides and lower the heat if the skin is beginning to burn. Cook for 15-20 minutes or until golden brown and crisp and cooked through. Serve right away.

44.Chicken and Vegetable Curry

Serves: 2

Ingredients:

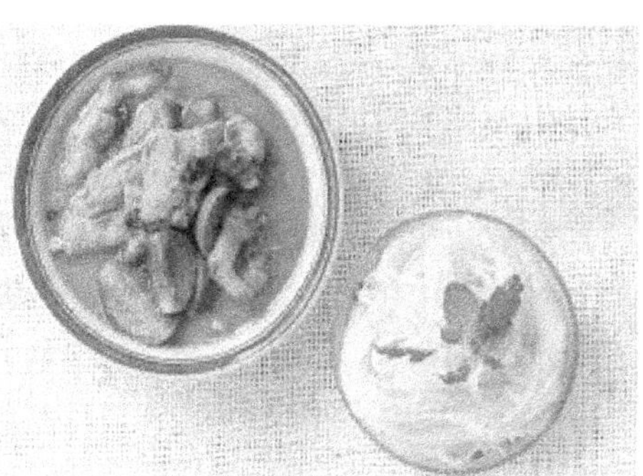

- ½ pound chicken thighs, boneless, chopped into bite sized pieces if desired
- 1 small yellow onion, chopped
- 4 ounces broccoli, cut into smaller florets
- 1 small red chili peppers, deseeded, chopped
- 1 3/4 ounces fresh green beans, chopped
- 1 ½ tbsp coconut oil or butter or more if required
- 1 can (14.5 ounce) coconut milk or coconut cream
- 2 tsp red curry paste or to taste
- 2 tsp fresh ginger, grated
- Cayenne pepper or to taste (optional)
- Salt to taste

Method:

1. Place a saucepan over medium heat. Add ghee or oil. When it heats, add onion, ginger and chili pepper and sauté until onions turn translucent.
2. Stir in the curry paste and chicken. Mix well.
3. Cook until chicken is light brown. Add more oil if necessary.
4. Add vegetables and the thick part of coconut cream and milk. Use the liquid in some other recipe like a smoothie. Cook until chicken and vegetables are tender.
5. Serve over rice.

45. Warm Chicken Salad
Serves: 4

Ingredients:

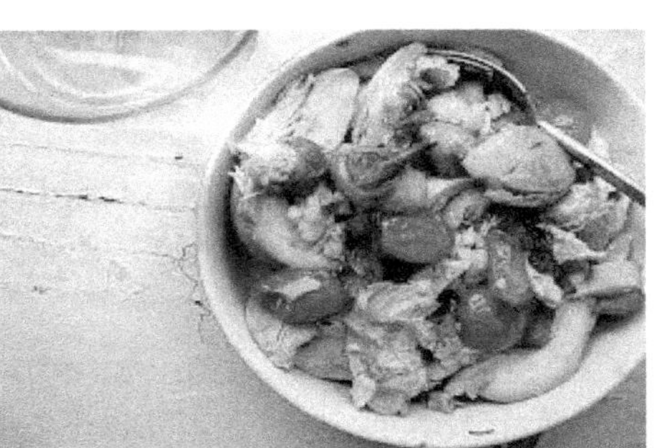

- 4 small chicken breasts, boneless, skinless, halved
- 2 large orange or red bell peppers, deseeded and cut into 1 inch squares
- 3 ½ ounces watercress, discard tough stalks
- 2/3 cucumber, sliced
- Juice of a small lemon
- Low calorie cooking oil spray
- 2 little gem lettuce leaves, separated
- 4 ripe medium tomatoes, chopped
- 2 tsp thick balsamic vinegar
- Sea salt to taste
- Freshly ground black pepper to taste

Method:

1. Sprinkle salt and pepper on both sides of the chicken.
2. Place a large nonstick pan over high heat. Spray cooking spray over it.
3. Add chicken and cook for 3 minutes. Flip sides and cook for 3 minutes or until tender inside. Remove with a slotted spoon and place on your cutting board. When cool enough to handle, slice the chicken.
4. Spray the pan with some more oil. Add peppers and sauté until slight blisters appear on the skin.
5. Divide and place lettuce leaves on 4 serving plates. Scatter watercress, cucumber, tomatoes and roasted peppers equally over it.
6. Divide and place chicken slices over the salad.
7. Trickle ½ tsp vinegar on each plate. Drizzle lemon juice on top. Sprinkle pepper on top and serve.

46.Chicken and Vegetable Balti

Serves: 4

Ingredients:

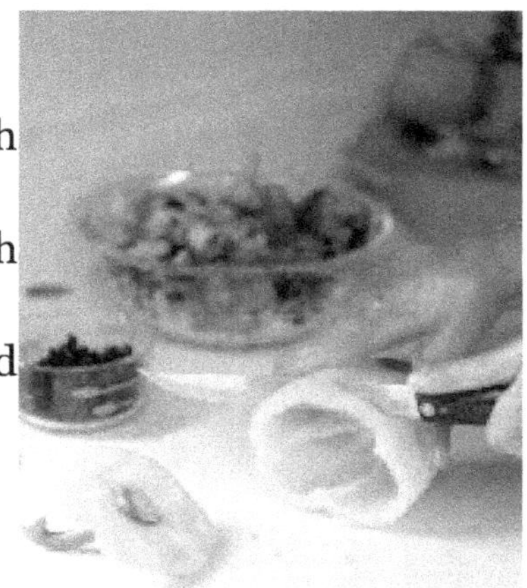

- 2 medium onions, thinly sliced
- 2 yellow bell peppers, deseeded, cut into 1 inch squares
- 2 red bell peppers, deseeded, cut into 1 inch squares
- 8 chicken thighs, boneless, skinless, trimmed of fat, cut each into 4 pieces
- 2 tbsp cornstarch
- 2 tbsp medium or mild curry powder
- 2 cans (8 ounces each) chopped tomatoes
- Freshly ground black pepper to taste
- 4 cloves garlic, peeled, thinly sliced
- 11 ounces fat free natural yogurt
- 1/3 cup fresh cilantro finely chopped + extra to garnish
- Low calorie cooking spray

Method:

1. Place a large deep nonstick frying pan or wok over medium heat. Spray some cooking spray and let the pan heat.
2. Sprinkle pepper over the chicken pieces.
3. Add onions into the pan and sauté until light brown.
4. Stir in the chicken and bell peppers. Sauté for 3-4 minutes. Flip sides after 2 minutes of cooking.
5. Add cornstarch, ¼ cup water and yogurt into a bowl. Whisk until well combined.
6. Dust the chicken with curry powder. Stir in the garlic and sauté for a minute or until fragrant.

7. Add tomatoes, yogurt mixture, 1-cup water and cilantro into a bowl and stir. Pour into the pan and stir constantly until it thickens.
8. Lower the heat and simmer until chicken is cooked through. Add some more pepper and stir.
9. Garnish with cilantro and serve.

47. Chicken Butternut Chili

Serves: 8

Ingredients:

- 2 tbsp canola oil
- 4 ribs celery, chopped
- 4 medium carrots, peeled, chopped
- 2 medium onions, chopped
- 2 medium tomatoes, chopped
- 4 cups butternut squash, peeled, cubed
- 4 tbsp tomato paste
- 4 cups chicken stock
- 2 envelopes low sodium chili seasoning mix
- 2 cups cooked, cubed chicken breast
- Salt to taste
- Pepper to taste
- A handful cilantro, chopped, to garnish

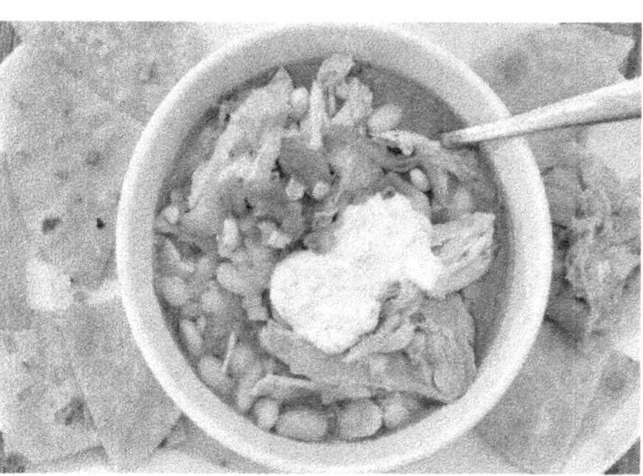

Method:

1. Place a soup pot over medium heat. Add oil. When the oil is heated, add carrots, onions and celery and sauté until onions are translucent.
2. Add butternut squash, tomato paste and tomatoes, seasoning mix and stock and stir.
3. When it begins to boil, lower the heat and simmer until squash is cooked.
4. Add chicken and heat thoroughly.
5. Ladle into bowls. Garnish with cilantro and serve.
6. Leftovers can be refrigerated or frozen.

48. Spicy Chicken and Spelt Salad

Serves: 5

Ingredients:

<u>For dressing:</u>

- 2 tbsp soy sauce
- 1 tbsp olive oil
- 1 ½ tbsp Asian sesame oil
- 1 tbsp rice wine vinegar
- A pinch cayenne pepper
- ½ tbsp garlic, grated
- ½ tbsp ginger, grated
- 1 tbsp creamy peanut butter
- ½ Serrano chili pepper, minced

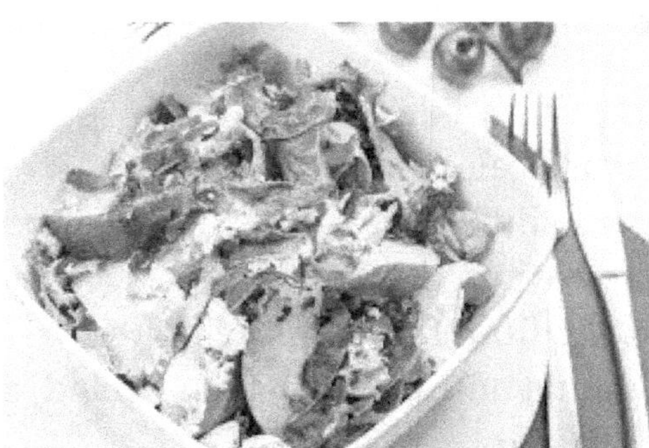

<u>For salad:</u>

- ½ cup spelt kernels
- ¼ tsp kosher salt
- 5 cups water, divided
- ¼ tsp salt
- 2 chicken breast halves, boneless
- ½ bunch green onions, thinly sliced
- 1 small onion, chopped into chunks
- ½ red bell pepper, sliced
- 2 tbsp cilantro, chopped
- 2 tbsp parsley, chopped
- 1 cup red cabbage, thinly sliced
- 2 carrots, thinly sliced

Method:

1. To make dressing: Add all the ingredients of dressing into a bowl and whisk well. Cover and set aside.
2. Place a skillet over medium high heat. Add spelt and roast until brown and a few would have popped. Transfer into a mesh strainer. Pour cold water over it and let it drain.
3. Add 3 cups water into a saucepan. Place saucepan over high heat. When it begins to boil, add kosher salt and spelt and stir. When it begins to boil again, lower the heat to low heat and cook until tender. It may take a long time. Drain and cool completely.
4. Place a skillet over high heat. Add 2 cups water. Add salt and onion. When it begins to boil, add chicken and lower the heat to medium. Cover and cook until chicken is done. Remove chicken from the pan and place on your cutting board. Use the broth in some other recipe or discard.
5.   When the chicken is cool enough to handle, chop into pieces and add into a large bowl.
6. Add rest of the ingredients and toss well. Pour dressing on top and toss well.

49.Spicy Cajun Chicken Quinoa

Serves: 2

Ingredients:

- 2 chicken breasts, cut into bite size pieces
- ¼ cup quinoa
- ¼ pouch (from a ½ pound pouch) ready to use Puy lentils
- 1 red onion, cut into thin wedges
- A handful fresh cilantro, chopped
- ½ tbsp Cajun seasoning
- 1 ¼ cups hot chicken stock
- ½ tbsp olive oil
- 1.8 ounces dried apricots, sliced
- ½ bunch spring onions

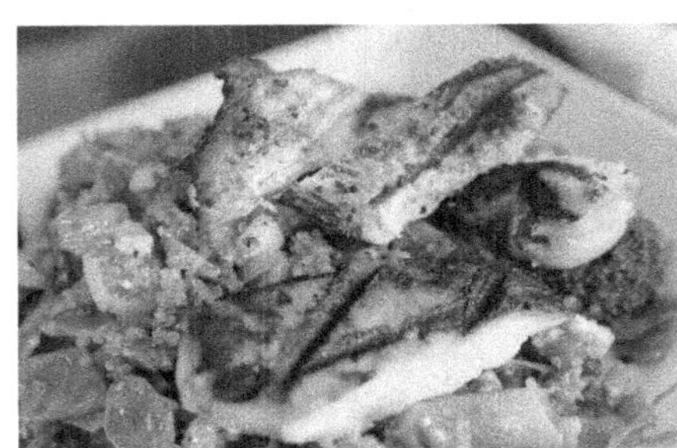

Method:

1. Sprinkle Cajun spice over the chicken and place in a baking pan.
2. Bake in a preheated oven at 390 ° F for 20 minutes or until done.
3. Meanwhile, add quinoa and stock into a saucepan. Place saucepan over medium heat. Cook until tender.
4. Add apricots and lentils during the last 5 minutes of cooking. Drain the excess water and add into a bowl. Add chicken and toss well.
5. Place a pan over medium heat. Add oil. When the oil is heated, add onion and sauté until translucent. Transfer into the bowl of quinoa. Add cilantro and spring onions and toss. Serve right away.

50.Moroccan Chicken & Lentils

Serves: 3

Ingredients:

- 1 cup carrots, chopped
- 1 pound chicken breast halves, skinless, boneless
- Salt to taste
- ¼ tsp ground cinnamon
- ¼ tsp ground cayenne
- ¾ cup dried lentils of your choice, rinsed
- 1 tbsp garlic, minced
- ½ tsp turmeric powder
- 2 cups fat free chicken broth

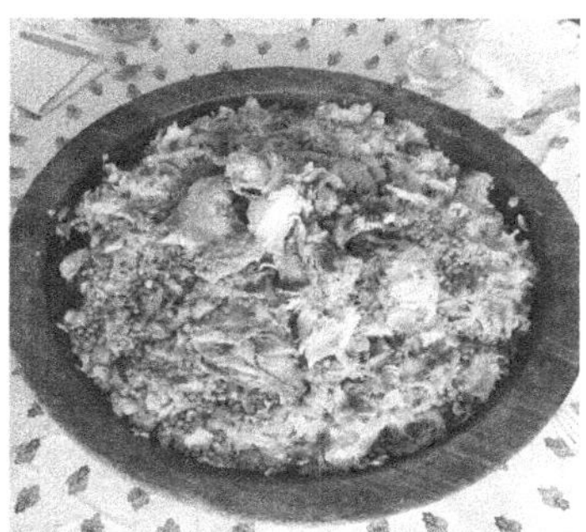

Method:

1. Add all the ingredients into a Dutch oven. Place Dutch oven over medium heat. When it begins to boil, lower the heat and simmer until chicken is tender.
2. Serve over rice.

51.Sweet Potato & Chicken with Gravy

Serves: 3

Ingredients:

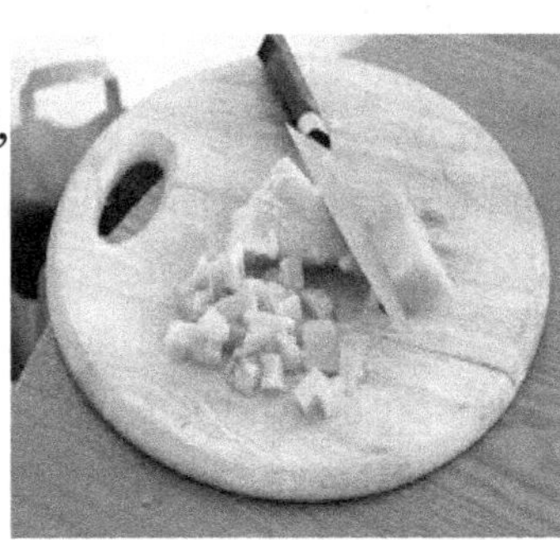

- 2 pounds chicken, skinless, boneless, chopped
- 10 ounces canned pineapple pieces, in juice
- 1 tbsp cornstarch mixed with 2 tbsp water
- 3 sweet potatoes, julienned
- 8 ounces chicken broth

Method:

1. Add chicken into a Dutch oven. Layer with sweet potatoes followed by pineapple. Pour broth over it. Cover and cook until chicken is tender.
2. Pour cornstarch mixture and stir constantly until thick.
3. Serve over rice or with bread.

52. Five Spice Chicken Wings

Serves: 4

Ingredients:

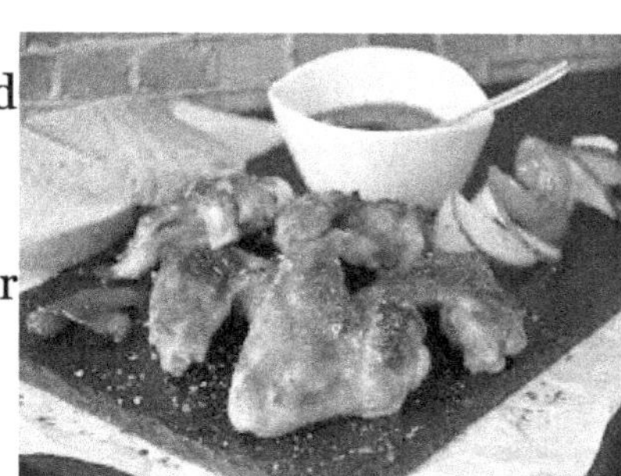

- 8 chicken wings, chop the wing tips and discard it, chop each into 2
- ½ tbsp butter, melted
- 6 tbsp plum sauce, unsweetened or sugar free
- ½ tsp five spice powder or to taste
- 1 green onion, thinly sliced, to garnish

Method:

1. Line a baking dish with foil. Spread wings in the dish.
2. Bake in a preheated oven at 390 ° F for 20 minutes. Drain liquid in the dish.
3. Mix together rest of the ingredients into a bowl and add into a pan. Add the chicken wings and stir well.
1. Heat thoroughly. Lower the heat and simmer for 5 minutes or until cooked.
2. Garnish with green onions and serve.

53. Mango Chicken Tacos

Serves: 8

Ingredients:

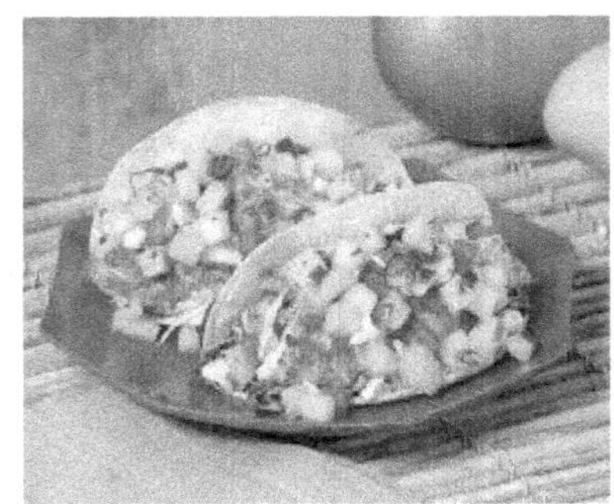

- 4 chicken breasts, boneless, skinless
- 1 cup low fat cheese, shredded
- 3 cups mango salsa
- Low fat sour cream, as required
- 8 whole wheat tortillas
- Lettuce as required, thinly sliced

Method:

1. Place Dutch oven over medium heat. Place the chicken in the pot. Pour mango salsa over the chicken and stir.
2. Cover and cook until tender.
3. Remove the chicken with a slotted spoon. When cool enough to handle, shred with a pair of forks and add it back to the pot. Mix well.
4. Spread tortillas on your countertop. Place chicken over the tortillas. Sprinkle lettuce and cheese and roll.
5. Serve right away.

54. Gingered Chutney Chicken

Serves: 4

Ingredients:

- 2 pounds chicken thighs
- 1/4 cup mango chutney or to taste
- 1 tbsp quick cooking tapioca mixed with a tbsp water
- 2-3 tbsp chili sauce
- 1 tsp fresh ginger, grated
- Salt to taste

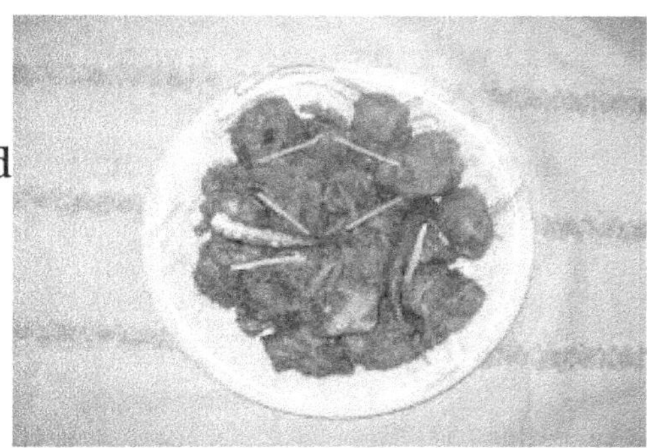

Method:

1. Place a Dutch oven over medium heat. Add all the ingredients into the pot. Mix well.
2. Cover and cook until chicken is tender.

55. Sesame Ginger Turkey Wraps

Serves: 4

Ingredients:

- 1 ½ -2 pounds turkey thighs, skinless
- 8 ounces broccoli slaw mix
- ½ cup bottled sesame ginger stir-fry sauce
- 3 green onions, thinly sliced
- 6 flour tortillas, warmed
- 2 tbsp water
- Cooking spray

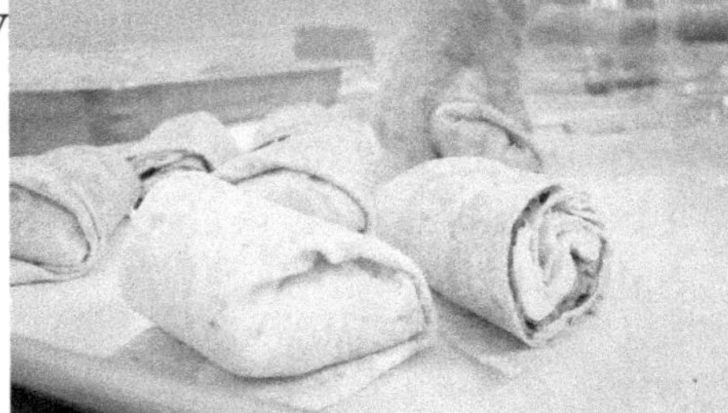

Method:

1. Place turkey breast in a Dutch oven.
2. Mix together water and sesame ginger stir fry sauce in a bowl and pour over the turkey breast.
3. Cover and cook until tender.
4. Remove the turkey with a slotted spoon and place on your cutting board. When cool enough to handle, shred the turkey with a pair of forks. Discard the bones. Add the turkey back to the pot and mix well.
5. Add broccoli slaw and stir. Cover and let it sit for 5 minutes.
6. Place tortillas on your countertop. Place the turkey slaw mixture on the tortillas. Garnish with green onions, wrap and serve.

56. Turkey and Avocado Lettuce Cups

Serves: 2

Ingredients:

- 8 ounces turkey, slices
- ½ avocado, peeled, pitted, sliced
- 8 butter lettuce leaves
- Salt to taste
- Pepper to taste

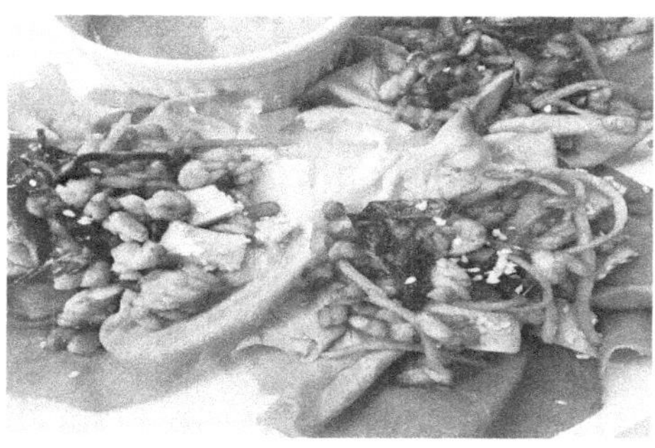

Method:

1. Place lettuce leaves on a serving platter.
2. Divide turkey slices and place on the lettuce leaves.
3. Divide the avocado slices and place on top of the turkey slices. Sprinkle salt and pepper on top.
4. Serve.

57. Turkey-Carrot Roll-Up

Serves: 2 (2 Roll-up each)

Ingredients:

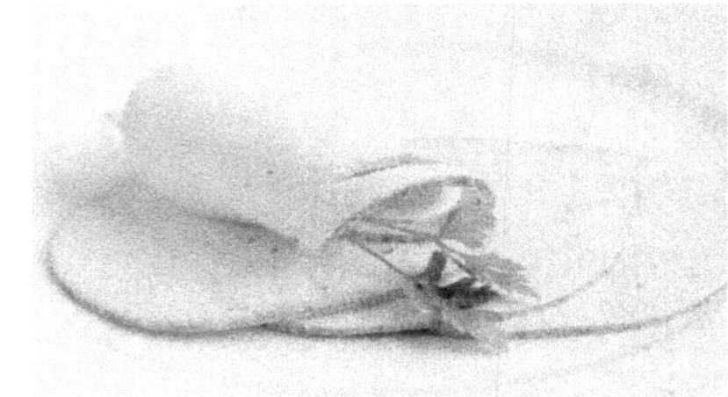

- 4 slices turkey breast
- 4 tsp yellow mustard
- 4 carrot sticks

Method:

1. Place turkey slices on a serving platter. Spread a tsp of mustard on each slice. Place a carrot stick on one end of the turkey slice. Roll and serve.

58. Pasta with Turkey and Broccoli

Serves: 8

Ingredients:

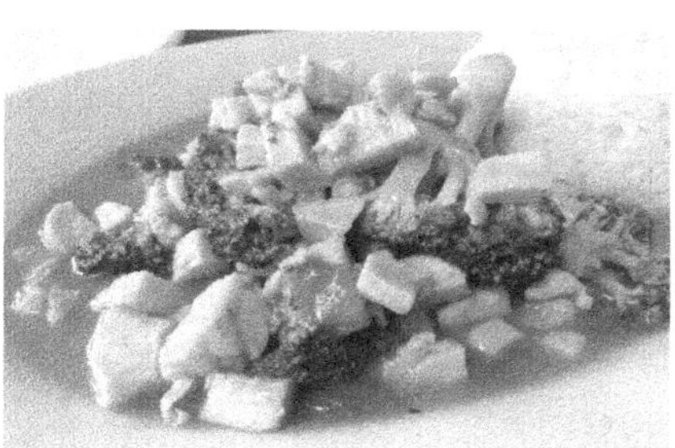

- 1 ½ pounds whole wheat Orecchiette
- 4 tbsp olive oil
- 4 cloves garlic, chopped
- 1 tsp crushed red pepper
- 4 cups broccoli florets
- 2 pounds ground turkey
- 2 tsp fennel seeds
- Low fat parmesan cheese to serve (optional)
- Kosher salt to taste

Method:

1. Follow the directions on the package and cook the pasta. Add broccoli a minute before turning off the heat. Drain and add pasta and broccoli into the saucepan.
2. Place a large skillet over medium high heat. Add 2 tbsp oil. When the oil is heated, add turkey, red pepper, fennel seeds and garlic. Cook until brown. Break the meat simultaneously as it cooks.
3. Add salt and stir. Add pasta mixture and 2 tbsp oil. Toss well and serve garnished with Parmesan.

59. Amaranth Fish Sticks

Serves: 4

Ingredients:

- 4 fish fillets, cut into sticks
- 2 eggs, beaten
- 1 cup amaranth
- 4-5 tbsp oil

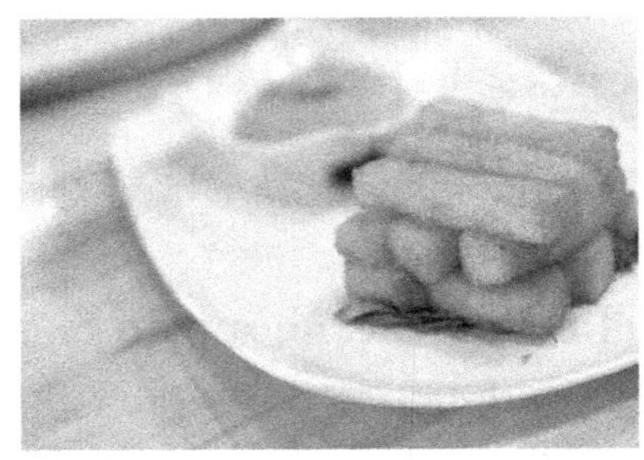

Method:

1. Place amaranth in a shallow bowl. Dip fish sticks in egg. Shake to drop off excess egg.
2. Dredge in amaranth and place on a plate.
3. Place a nonstick pan over medium heat. Add 2-3 tbsp oil. Place half the sticks on the pan and cook until golden brown. Flip sides and cook the other side until golden brown.
4. Repeat the previous step with the remaining fish sticks.

60. Summer Garden Fish Tacos

Serves: 8

Ingredients:

- 2 medium ears sweet corn, husk removed, chopped
- 8 tilapia fillets (4 ounces each) grilled or baked
- 2 yellow summer squashes, halved lengthwise, chopped
- 1 large red onion, chopped
- 2 tsp lime zest, grated
- 16 whole wheat tortillas, warmed
- 2 poblano peppers, halved, deseeded
- ¼ tsp salt
- 2 medium heirloom tomatoes, chopped
- 1/3 cup fresh cilantro, chopped
- 1/3 cup lime juice
- 1 medium ripe avocado, peeled, sliced

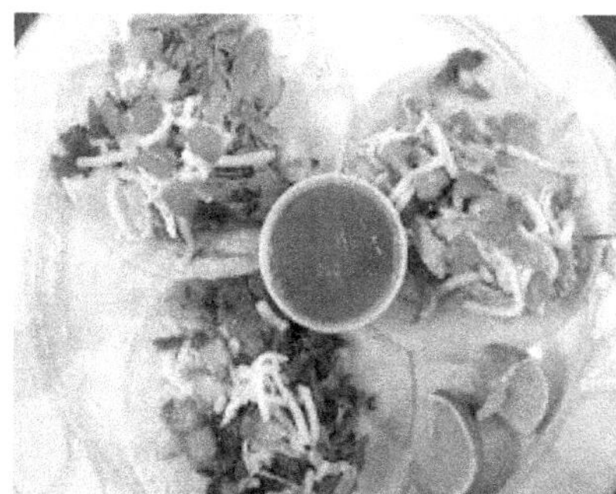

Method:

1. Place a fillet over each tortilla.
2. Add corn, pepper, squash, tomato, onion, lime juice, cilantro and lime zest into a bowl. Mix well.
3. Place vegetable mixture over the fillets. Fold over and serve.

61. Crisp Mashed Potato Fish Cakes

Serves: 7-8

Ingredients:

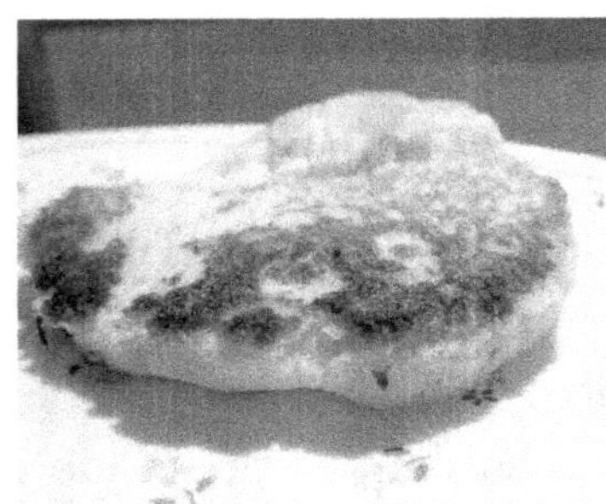

- 5 cups fresh or leftover mashed potatoes
- 2 eggs
- 4 cups whole wheat panko breadcrumbs
- 3 cups cooked fish, shredded
- 1 tsp cracked pepper
- Paprika to taste
- 3 cups cooked fish, shredded
- ½ cup low fat parmesan cheese, grated
- Salt to taste (optional)
- Oil, as required, to fry

Method:

1. Add mashed potatoes and fish into a bowl and mash well. Add egg, panko breadcrumbs, cracked pepper, paprika, cheese and salt and mix until well combined.
2. Divide the mixture into 7-8 equal portions and shape into patties.
3. Place a skillet over medium heat. Add 3-4 tbsp oil. When the oil is heated, place 3-4 patties in the pan. Cook until the underside is golden brown. Flip sides and cook the other side until golden brown.
4. Follow the previous step and cook the remaining cakes.
5. Serve with a dip of your choice.

62.Salmon, Black Bean, and Corn Tostadas

Serves: 2

Ingredients:

- 2 cooked salmon fillets (skinless), skinless, flaked into pieces
- 8 tostada shells
- 2 cups fresh corn
- 1 cup salsa Verde
- 2 cups canned or cooked black beans, rinsed
- 3 cups romaine lettuce, shredded
- 2 limes, cut into wedges, to serve
- Salt to taste
- Pepper to taste

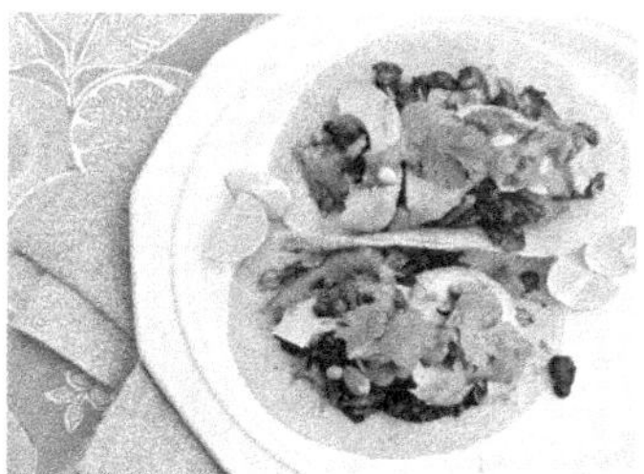

Method:

1. Place a tostada shell on each of 8 serving plates. Divide equally the corn, black beans, and lettuce over the tostada shells. Scatter salmon all over. Sprinkle salt and pepper. Drizzle 2 tbsps salsa on each.
2. Serve along with lime wedges.

63. Red Mullet with Baked Tomatoes

Serves: 8

Ingredients:

<u>For tomatoes:</u>

- 26 ounces mixed red and yellow cherry tomatoes
- 4 cloves garlic, minced
- Low calorie cooking spray
- 23 ounces fine green beans, trimmed
- 4 tbsp lemon juice
- Salt to taste
- Freshly ground pepper to taste

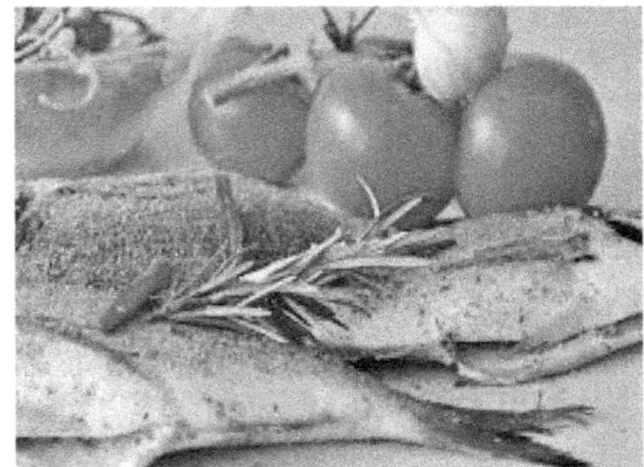

<u>For red mullet:</u>

- 16 red mullet fillets
- 4 tsp baby capers, drained
- Zest of 2 lemons, finely grated
- 4 spring onions, finely sliced
- Salt to taste
- Freshly ground pepper to taste
-

<u>For garnishing:</u>

- 16 capers
- ¼ cup parsley, chopped

Method:

1. Add all the ingredients for tomatoes into a baking dish and toss. Spray with cooking spray.
2. Bake in a preheated oven at 390 ° F for 10 minutes.
3. Take 8 large sheets of foil and line with similar size baking paper.

4. Lay 2 fillets on the center of each sheet. Sprinkle rest of the ingredients for mullet over the fillets.
5. Fold the sides of the foil over the filling. Press the edges to seal.
6. Place the foil packets on a large baking sheet. Place the baking next beside the baking dish. Bake for 10 minutes or until the fish flakes easily when pricked with a fork.
7. Divide the vegetables into 8 portions. Serve one fish packet with each portion of vegetables, garnished with capers and parsley.

64.Sheet Pan Salmon with Kale, Orange, and Farro

Serves: 2

Ingredients:

- 2 medium oranges, peeled, separated into segments, chopped
- Salt to taste
- Pepper to taste
- 2 salmon fillets (4 ounces each) discard skin
- 2 tbsp canola oil
- 2 cups kale leaves, discard hard stems and ribs, thinly sliced
- 1 ½ cups cooked farro, warmed

Method:

1. Place a sheet of parchment paper over a rimmed baking sheet.
2. Add oranges into a bowl along with any juice while chopping. Add oil, salt and pepper and stir. Add kale and stir. Transfer on to the prepared baking sheet.
3. Sprinkle salt and pepper generously over the salmon on both the sides and place over the kale.
4. Bake in a preheated oven at 450 ° F for 7-10 minutes or until the way you like it cooked but remove the kale and oranges from the pan if you want salmon cooked for more than 10 minutes.
5. Divide farro between 2 plates. Place kale and orange mixture over it. Top with salmon and serve.

65. Roasted Cod with Orange & Radicchio

Serves: 2

Ingredients:

- 2 cod fillets (5 ounces each), boneless, skinless
- ½ head radicchio, torn
- A handful flat leaf parsley, chopped
- 2 tbsp olive oil
- 1 orange, cut into segments
- 1 tsp orange zest
- 2 tbsp orange juice

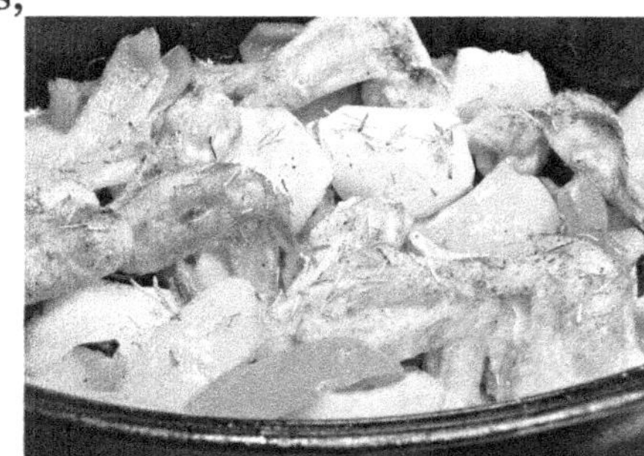

Method:

1. Place fillets on a rimmed baking sheet. Brush with oil.
2. Bake in a preheated oven at 400 ° F for 7-10 minutes or until it flakes easily.
3. Add rest of the ingredients into a bowl and toss.
4. Divide the salad into 2 plates. Place a fillet on each plate and serve.

66. Lemon-Tarragon Shrimp Pasta

Serves: 2

Ingredients:

- ½ pound shrimp, tail-on, peeled, deveined
- 6 ounces whole wheat linguine
- ¼ cup cooked water
- 1 tbsp fresh tarragon, chopped
- ¼ cup olive oil
- 1 tbsp lemon juice
- ¾ tsp lemon zest, grated
- Salt to taste
- Pepper to taste

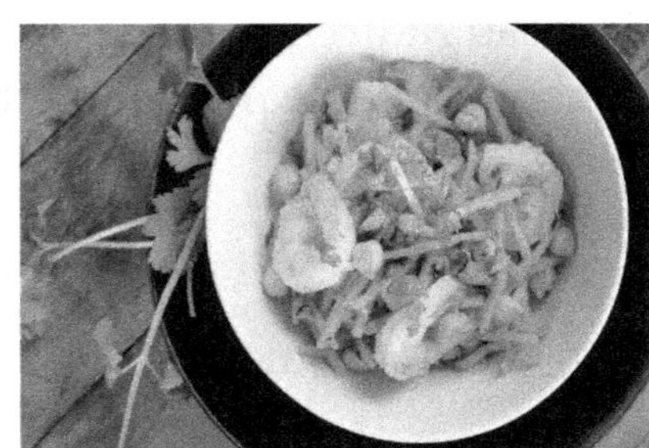

Method:

1. Cook linguine following the instructions on the package. Drain and retained ¼ cup of the cooked liquid.
2. Place a skillet over medium high heat. Add oil. When the oil is heated, add shrimp and sauté for 3 minutes or until done.
3. Add rest of the ingredients and toss well. Heat thoroughly and serve.

67. Black Bean Soup

Serves: 2

Ingredients:

- 1 ½ cans (15 ounces each) black beans, with its liquid
- ¼ cup fresh cilantro + extra to garnish
- 1 clove garlic, minced
- ½ pound good quality salsa
- 1 tsp ground cumin

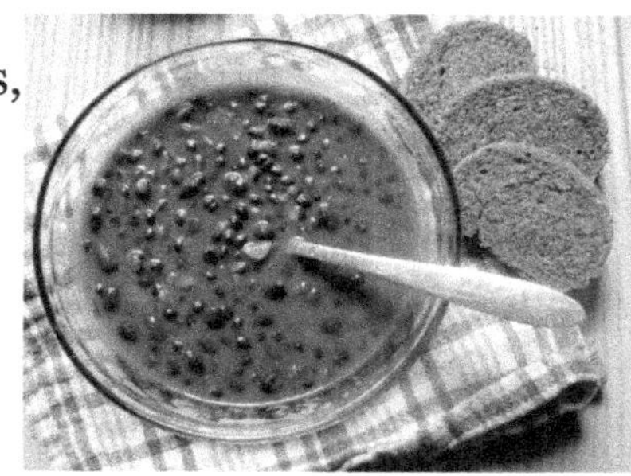

Method:

1. Place a saucepan over medium high heat. Add all the ingredients into it and stir. When it begins to boil, lower the heat and simmer for 5-7 minutes.
2. Ladle into soup bowls. Garnish with cilantro and serve.

68. Black-Eyed Pea Salad

Serves: 2

Ingredients:

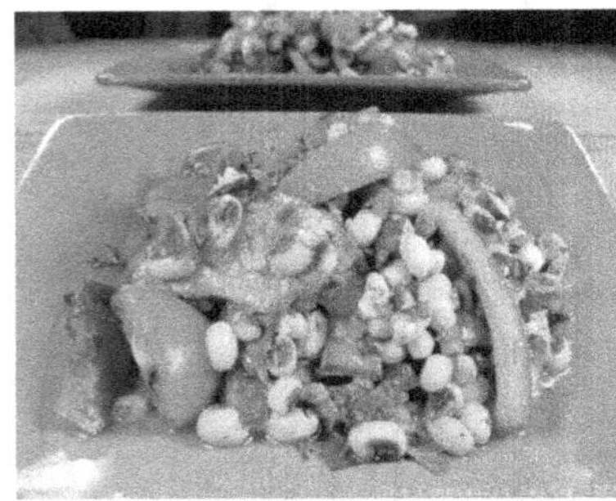

- ½ cup grape tomatoes, halved
- 1 tbsp red wine vinegar
- Pepper to taste
- 1 cup baby arugula
- 1 ¼ tbsp canola mayonnaise
- ¼ tsp kosher salt or to taste
- ½ can (from a 15 ounces can) black eyed peas, unsalted, rinsed, drained

Method:

1. Add all the ingredients into a bowl and toss well.

69. Hearty Vegetable Soup

Serves: 4

Ingredients:

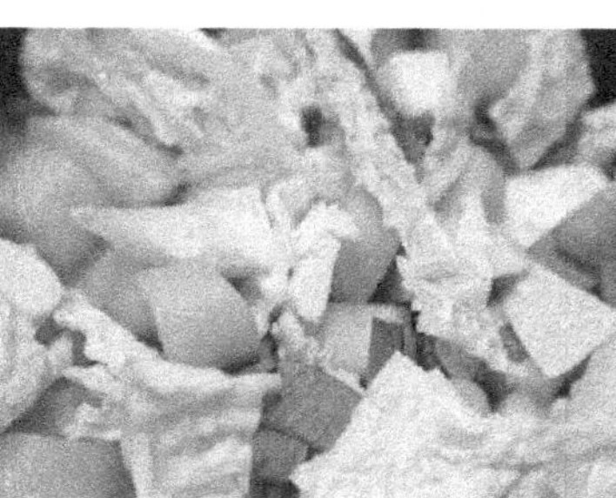

- 2 medium onions, sliced
- 4 celery sticks, trimmed, thinly sliced
- 2 cans (14 ounces each) chopped tomatoes
- 2 tsp dried mixed herbs
- 2 heads (4 ½ ounces) young spring greens, trimmed, sliced
- Low calorie cooking spray
- 4 cloves garlic, thinly sliced
- 2 medium carrots, chopped into 1 inch pieces
- 2 medium yellow bell peppers, chopped into 1 inch squares
- 2 vegetable stock cubes, crumbled
- 2 cans (14 ounces each) butter beans, drained, rinsed
- Sea salt to taste
- Freshly ground pepper to taste

Method:

1. Place a large nonstick pan or pot over medium heat. Spray some cooking spray in the pan.
2. Add celery, onion, garlic, carrot and bell pepper and sauté and until tender.
3. Add tomatoes, water, stock cubes and herbs and stir. When it begins to boil, lower the heat and simmer for 20-30 minutes.
4. Add salt, pepper, butter beans and spring greens and simmer for 5 minutes.
5. Ladle into bowls and serve.

70. Chermoula Tofu and Roasted Red Vegetables

Serves: 8

Ingredients:

For chermoula tofu:

- A large handful fresh cilantro, finely chopped
- 2 tsp cumin seeds, lightly crushed
- 1 tsp dried crushed chilies
- 18 ounces tofu
- 6 cloves garlic, chopped
- Zest of 2 lemons, finely grated
- 2 tbsp olive oil

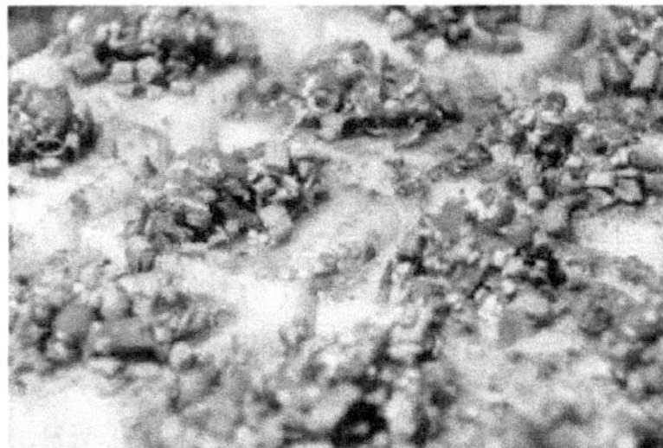

For roasted vegetables:

- 4 red onions, quartered
- 4 yellow bell pepper, deseeded
- 4 red pepper, deseeded, sliced
- 4 courgette, thickly sliced
- A pinch salt
- 2 small eggplants, thickly sliced
- Low calorie cooking spray

Method:

1. <u>To make chermoula:</u> Add cilantro, cumin, dried chili, garlic, zest and olive oil into a bowl and mix well.
2. Dry tofu by patting with paper towels. Cut each into 2 halves. Cut each half into thin slices horizontally.
3. Spread a liberal amount of this mixture over the tofu slices.
4. <u>To make roasted vegetables:</u> Spread the vegetables in a baking pan. Spray some cooking spray over the vegetables and toss well.

5. Bake in a preheated oven at 390 °F for 45 minutes or until slightly charred. Flip the vegetables a couple of times while baking.
6. Place the tofu slices over the vegetables with the chermoula side facing up. Bake for another 10-15 minutes.
7. Divide the tofu slices along with the roasted vegetables into 8 plates and serve.

71. Vegetables with Red Pepper Rouille

Serves: 3

Ingredients:

<u>For vegetables:</u>

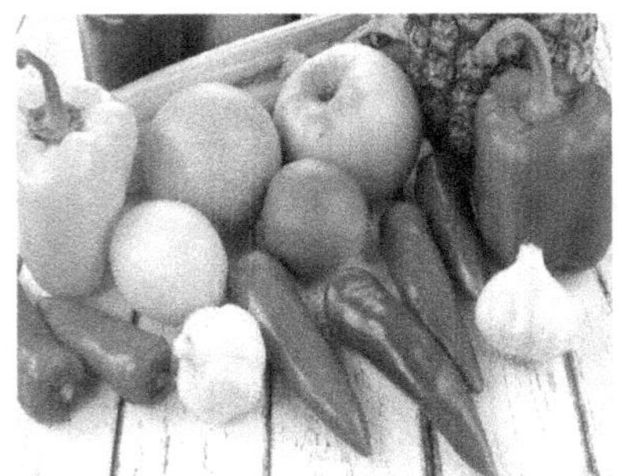

- 2 tbsp olive oil
- 2 pinches saffron threads
- 1 ½ courgettes, cut into 1 inch chunks
- Salt to taste
- Freshly ground black pepper
- 1 -2 cloves garlic, finely chopped
- 1 red bell pepper, cut into 6 strips
- 1 orange bell pepper, cut into 6 strips
- 1 onion, cut into wedges

<u>For rouille:</u>

- 4.5 ounces plum tomatoes
- 1 clove garlic, finely chopped
- ½ tbsp olive oil
- ½ red pepper, cored, cut into 1 inch squares
- Ground smoked paprika to taste

Method:

1. Add all the ingredients for vegetables into a Ziploc bag and seal the bag. Shake the ingredients until well coated. Let it marinate for 30 minutes.
2. <u>To make rouille:</u> Add tomatoes into a baking pan. Sprinkle garlic, pepper, salt and paprika over it. Trickle oil over the tomatoes.
3. Bake in a preheated oven at 430 °F for 15 minutes. Remove from the oven and cool. Peel the skin of the tomatoes and pepper. Add into a blender and blend until smooth. Pour into a bowl. Cover and keep warm.

4. Empty the contents of the Ziploc bag into a baking pan. Bake for 15-20 minutes or until brown. Turn the vegetables halfway through baking.
5. Divide the vegetables into 3 plates. Divide the rouille among the plates and serve.

72. Caponata Ratatouille

Serves: 3

Ingredients:

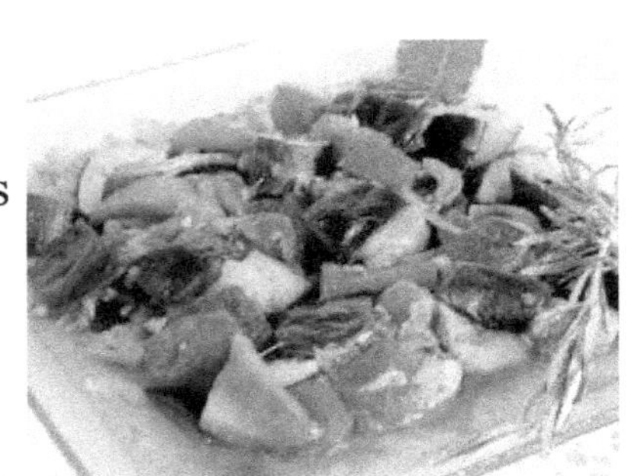

- ½ tbsp olive oil
- 1 medium onion, cut into 1 ½ inch chunks
- 1 large beef tomatoes, peeled, deseeded
- ¼ tsp cayenne pepper
- 1 tbsp pitted green olives
- 1 tbsp cocoa powder (optional)
- 5 ounces eggplant, cut into 1 ½ inch chunks
- 2 celery sticks, chopped
- ½ tsp chopped fresh thyme
- 1 tbsp capers, drained
- 2 tbsp white vinegar
- Freshly ground pepper to taste
- A handful fresh parsley, chopped, to garnish
- 5-6 almonds, chopped, to garnish

Method:

1. Place a nonstick pan over medium heat. Add oil. When the oil is very hot, add eggplant and cook until soft. Sprinkle some boiling water if necessary if the eggplant is getting stuck to the pan.
2. Place a skillet over medium heat. Add onion, celery and a couple of tbsp of water and cook for a few minutes until slightly tender.
3. Add tomatoes, cayenne pepper, thyme and eggplant and stir. Lower the heat and cook for 7-8 minutes.
4. Add rest of the ingredients and stir. Simmer for a couple of minutes.
5. Serve in bowls garnished with parsley and almonds.

73. No Cheese Quesadillas

Serves: 6

Ingredients:

- Extra chunky salsa, as required
- 12 yellow no oil corn tortillas
- 2 medium onions, chopped
- 1 small yellow bell pepper, chopped
- 1 small green bell pepper, chopped
- 1 small red bell pepper, chopped
- 1 ½ cups no oil refried pinto beans
- Chili powder, to taste

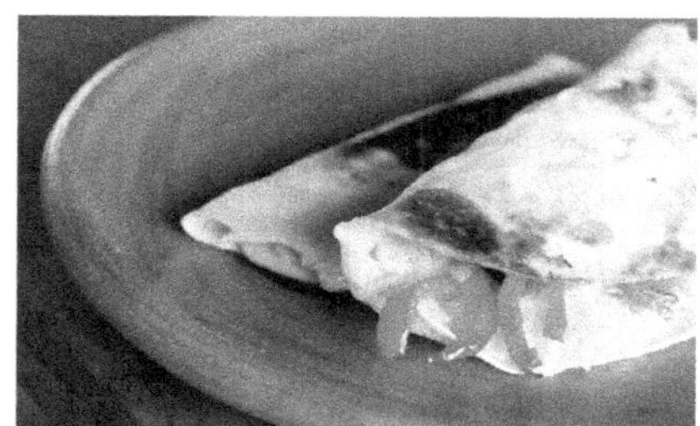

Method:

1. Place a tortilla on your countertop. Spread 4 tbsp refried beans over it.
2. Sprinkle a little of onions, bell peppers and chili powder over it.
3. Cover with another tortilla.
4. Place a nonstick pan over medium heat. Carefully lift the quesadilla and place on the pan. Cook until the underside is crisp. Flip sides and cook the other side until crisp.
5. Repeat steps 1-4 to make remaining quesadillas.
6. Cut each into 4 wedges and serve with salsa.

74. Pea and Farro Stir-Fry

Serves: 2-3

Ingredients:

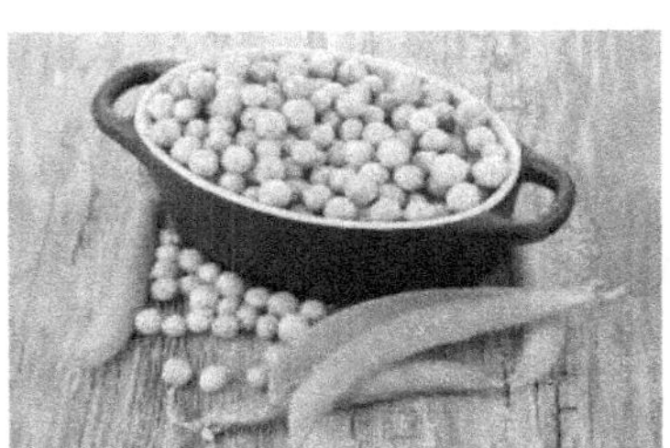

- 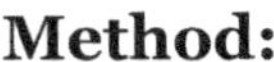 ½ cup fresh basil, torn
- ½ tsp paprika
- 2 cups fresh or frozen peas, thaw if frozen
- 1 1/3 cups cooked farro
- Pepper to taste
- Salt to taste
- 4 cloves garlic, minced
- 1 medium sweet onion, thinly sliced
- 4 large eggs, beaten
- 4 tsp olive oil, divided

Method:

1. Place a large cast iron skillet over medium high heat. Add 2 tsp oil. When the oil is heated, crack the eggs and stir constantly until scrambled and cooked.
2. Add garlic, pepper and salt and sauté until aromatic.
3. Stir in the rest of the ingredients and heat thoroughly.

75. Kamut Savory Salad

Serves: 4-5

Ingredients:

- 1 cup kamut grain, soaked in water overnight, drained
- ¼ cup frozen mixed vegetables
- 1 small carrot, chopped
- ½ cup mixed bell pepper, chopped
- 1 small onion, chopped
- ¼ cup canned or cooked red kidney beans
- 1 tsp olive oil
- 3 cups vegetable stock
- Salt to taste
- Pepper to taste
- Spring onion, to garnish
- Parsley, to garnish

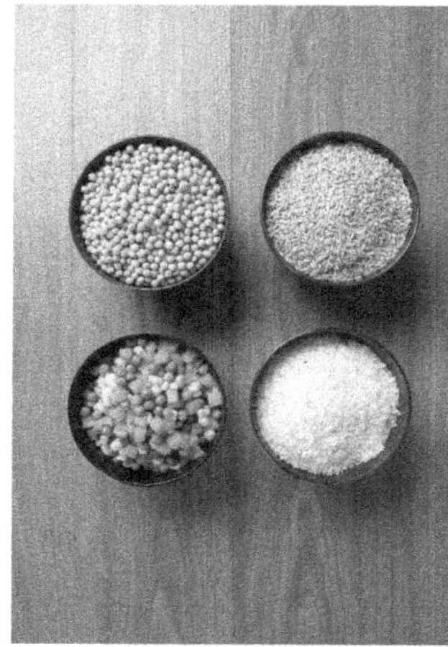

Method:

1. Add kamut and stock into a saucepan. Place a saucepan over medium heat. Cook until tender. Set aside.
2. Place a pan over medium heat. Add oil. When the oil is heated, add onion and sauté until translucent.
3. Add rest of the ingredients and stir. Heat thoroughly.
4. Sprinkle spring onions and parsley and serve.

76. Freekeh Salad

Serves: 2-3

Ingredients:

- 2 vine tomatoes, chopped or 4 cherry tomatoes, quartered
- Sea salt to taste
- 2 tbsp olive oil
- Juice of ½ lemon
- Zest of ½ lemon, grated
- A handful fresh cilantro or parsley, chopped
- 1 small cucumber, chopped
- ½ cup corn kernels
- 1 small onion, chopped
- ¾ cup freekeh
- 2 cups water

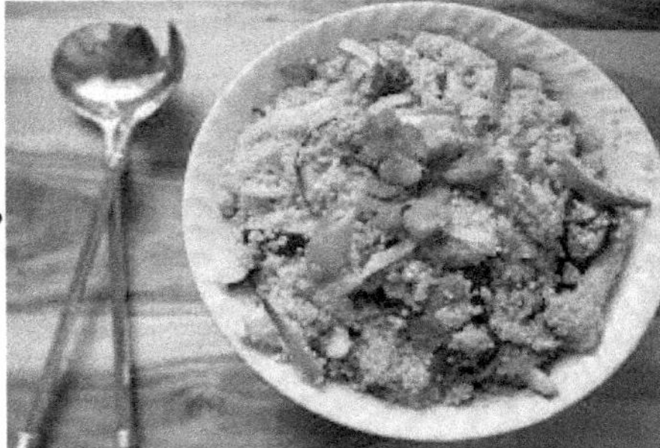

To serve:

- Hummus or pesto as required
- Avocado slices
- Mini tortillas or wraps, as required

Method:

1. Add freekeh and water. Place water over medium heat. When it begins to boil, lower the heat and cover with a lid. Simmer for 10-12 minutes. Uncover and cook until tender. Drain and set aside.
2. Add lemon juice, oil, zest, salt and pepper into a small bowl and whisk well.
3. Add rest of the ingredients including freekeh into a bowl and toss well. Pour dressing on top and toss well. Chill until ready to use.

4. Spread tortillas on your countertop. Place salad on one half of the tortillas. Top with avocado and hummus. Fold the other half over the filling and serve.

77. Kamut, Lentil, and Chickpea Soup

Serves: 8-10

Ingredients:

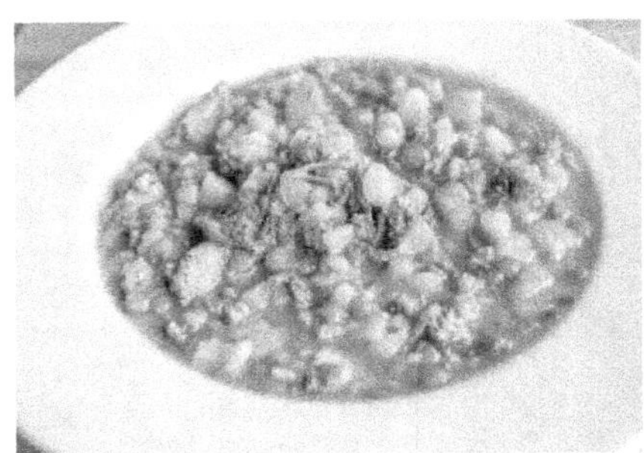

- 1 ½ cups kamut berries, rinsed
- 4 tbsp olive oil
- 2 cups carrots, finely chopped
- 1 cup celery, thinly sliced
- 4 tsp fresh thyme, chopped
- 4 cloves garlic, minced
- 4 bay leaves
- ½ tsp pepper powder
- A handful celery leaves, chopped (optional)
- 4 cups boiling water
- 4 cups onion, finely chopped
- 1 ½ cups fresh parsley, chopped
- 2 tbsp chopped fresh thyme
- 8 cans (14.5 ounces each) chicken broth or use equivalent homemade broth
- 2/3 cup dried lentils, rinsed, soaked in water for 20 minutes
- 2 cans (15 ounces each) chickpeas, rinsed, drained

Method:

1. Add kamut into a bowl. Cover with boiling water. Let it soak for 30 minutes.
2. Place a soup pot over medium heat. Add oil. When the oil is heated, add onion and herbs and sauté until onions are translucent.
3. Add garlic and saute until fragrant.
4. Add rest of the ingredients except chickpeas and stir. Cover and cook until tender.
5. Ladle into soup bowls. Sprinkle celery and serve.

78. Amaranth and Quinoa Stuffed Peppers

Serves: 8

Ingredients:

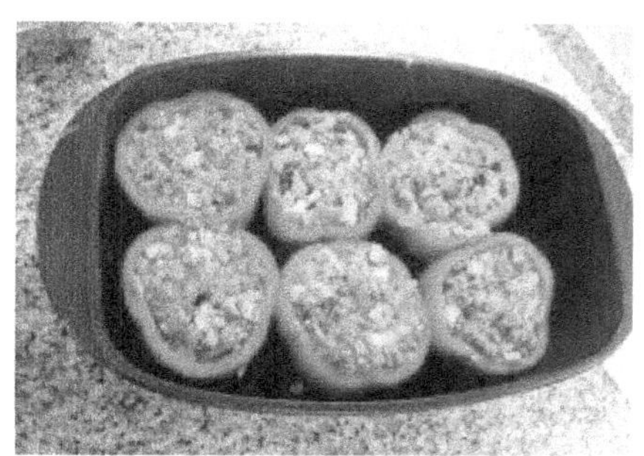

- 1 cup amaranth
- 1 cup black quinoa
- 2 cups edamame, cooked
- 4 shallots, chopped
- 2 carrots, grated
- 4 tbsp sesame seeds
- Salt to taste
- Pepper to taste
- 4 tbsp brown rice vinegar
- 8 bell peppers, slice off the tops

Method:

1. Cook quinoa and amaranth following the directions on the package.
2. Add into a bowl. Set aside the bell peppers and add rest of the ingredients into the bowl and stir.
3. Fill this mixture into the bell peppers. Place in a baking dish. Pour ½ cup water round the bell peppers.
4. Cover the dish with foil.
5. Bake in a preheated oven at 350 °F for 40-50 minutes or until done.

79. Black Bean Burritos

Serves: 4

Ingredients:

- 1 yam, cut into bite size pieces, steamed
- Low calorie cooking spray
- 1 small onion, chopped
- ¼ cup red bell pepper, chopped
- 1 jalapeño pepper, chopped
- 1 clove garlic, chopped
- 1 tomato, chopped
- 1 cup cooked or canned black beans
- ½ cup salsa
- 1 tbsp lime juice
- A handful fresh cilantro, chopped
- ½ cup cooked amaranth
- ½ tsp ground cumin
- ½ tsp chili powder
- Whole wheat tortillas to serve

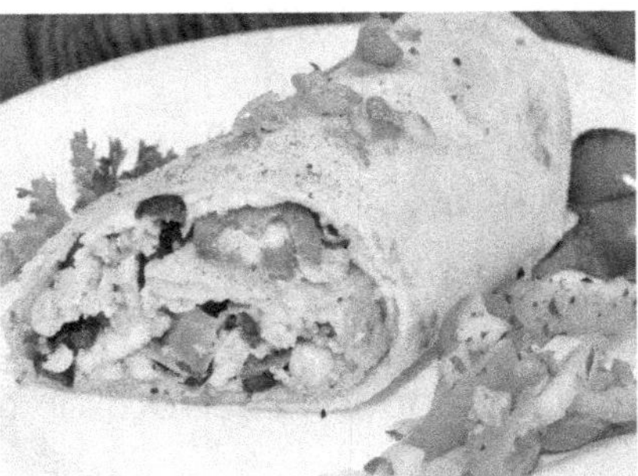

Method:

1. Place a nonstick skillet over medium heat. Spray with cooking spray.
2. Add onion, jalapeño pepper and bell pepper and sauté until onions are translucent.
3. Add garlic and sauté until fragrant. Add yam, salsa, cilantro, tomatoes, beans and lime juice and stir. Cook for 2-3 minutes.
4. Add spices and stir.
5. Serve over tortillas. Wrap like a burrito and serve.

80. Amaranth Risotto

Serves: 2

Ingredients:

- 1 tbsp olive oil, divided
- 1 tbsp butter, divided
- 1 medium yellow onion, chopped
- ½ cup porcini mushrooms
- 1 cup boiling hot water
- 2 cloves garlic, sliced
- ½ pound mushrooms of your choice
- 1 cup amaranth
- 1 ¼ cups cold water
- ½ tbsp soy sauce
- 1 ½ tbsp sherry
- Salt to taste

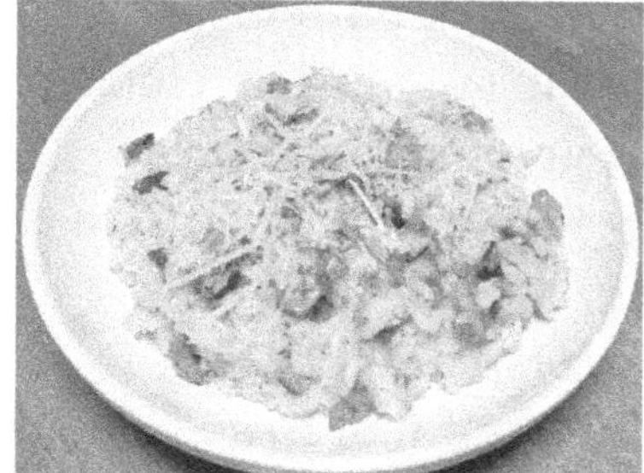

Method:

1. Add porcini mushrooms into a bowl. Pour boiling hot water over it. After 15 minutes, drain the water and retain the drained water. Squeeze the water from mushrooms. Chop into smaller pieces and set aside.
2. Place a pot over low heat. Add ½ tbsp butter and ½ tbsp oil. When butter melts, add onion and sauté until translucent. Add the retained water, cold water and amaranth and stir. Cover and allow it to boil.
3. Lower the heat and simmer until amaranth is tender. Add salt and stir. Turn off the heat.
4. Place a skillet over medium heat. Add remaining oil and butter. When it is heated, add garlic and both the mushrooms and sauté for a couple of minutes.
5. Add salt and soy sauce and cook until tender. Add sherry and cook for a couple of minutes. Remove from heat.
6. Serve mushrooms over risotto.

81. Herby Rice

Serves: 3

Ingredients:

- 1 ¼ cups + 2 tbsp converted long grain rice
- 1 ½ tbsp butter
- 1 can (14 ounces) chicken broth
- 3 green onions, sliced
- 3 tbsp pine nuts, toasted
- ½ tsp salt or to taste
- ½ tsp dried basil
- A handful of fresh basil, chopped to garnish

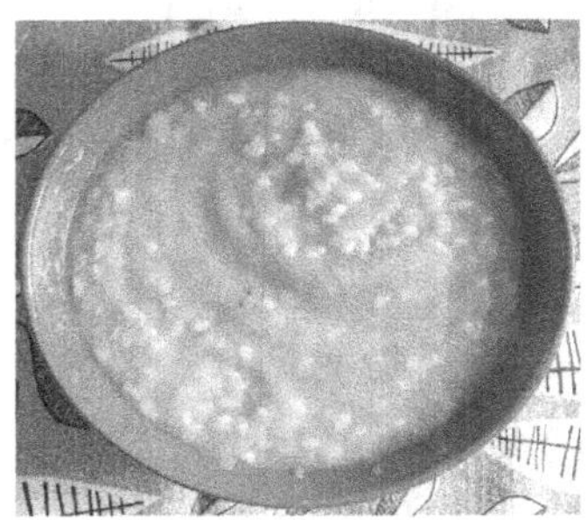

Method:

1. Place a large skillet over medium heat. Add butter and rice and sauté until golden brown.
2. Add rest of the ingredients except pine nuts and basil and stir.
3. Cover and cook until rice is tender and moisture absorbed. When done, fluff with a fork.
4. Add pine nuts and stir.
5. Garnish with basil and serve.

Chapter Three: Occasional Treats

82.Strawberry Crème Truffles

Serves: 15-20

Ingredients:

For filling:

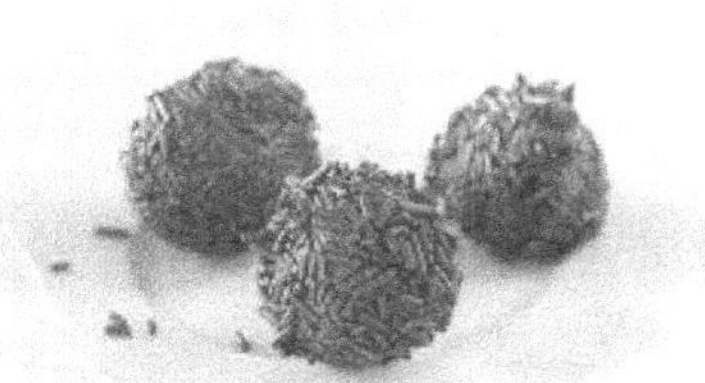

- 2 tbsp swerve sweetener or stevia powder to taste
- 2 cups strawberries, sliced
- 2 cups coconut butter

For chocolate:

- 6 tbsp almond milk or milk of your choice
- 2 cups dark chocolate chips (stevia sweetened)

Method:

1. To make filling: Add all the ingredients of filling into a food processor and process until well combined.
2. Line a baking sheet with parchment paper. Remove small scoops of the mixture and drop on the prepared baking sheet. If the mixture is too soft, chill for a few minutes until you are able to scoop.
3. Place the baking sheet in the freezer until set.
4. Meanwhile, add chocolate chips and milk into a heatproof container. Place on a double boiler and melt the chocolate. Stir frequently.
5. Drop the firm balls into the chocolate. Carefully lift with a pair of forks and place them on the baking sheet.
6. Place in the freezer until the chocolate is firm.

83.Instant Avocado Vanilla Pudding

Serves: 8 -10

Ingredients:

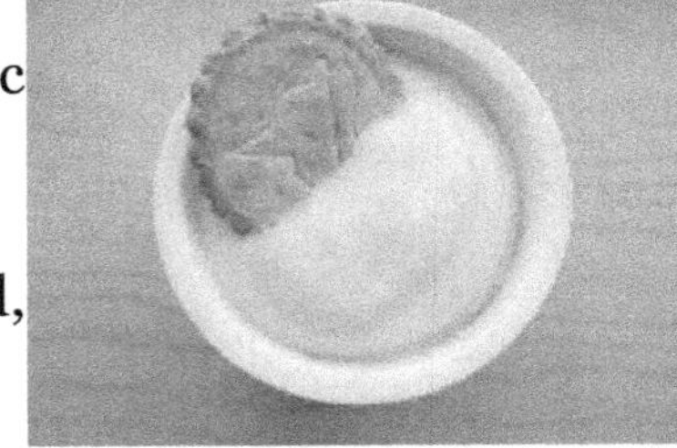

- 2 cans (14.5 ounces each) organic coconut milk, chilled
- Liquid stevia drops to taste
- 4 ripe Hass avocados, peeled, pitted, chopped
- 4 tsp vanilla extract
- 2 tbsp fresh lime juice

Method:

1. Gather all the ingredients and add into a blender. Blend until smooth and thick.
2. Pour into 8-10 bowls.
3. Chill if desired and serve.

84. Peanut Butter Banana Ice Cream

Serves: 4

Ingredients:

- 4 ripe bananas, sliced, frozen
- A handful roasted peanuts, chopped
- 2 tbsp creamy peanut butter

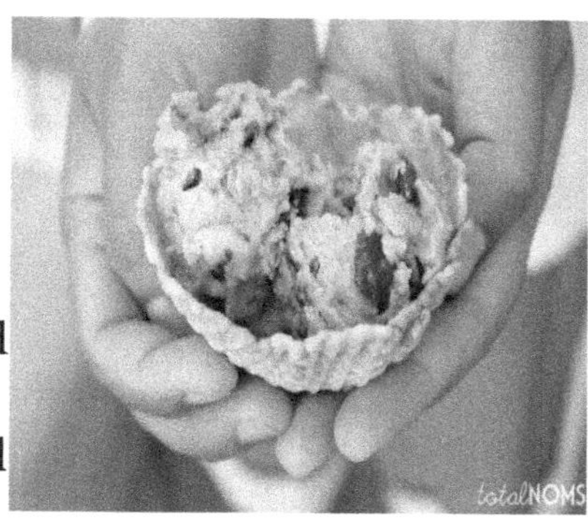

Method:

1. Add frozen banana into a blender and blend until smooth.
2. Add peanut butter and blend until well combined.
3. Serve right away or freeze and serve later.
4. Garnish with peanuts while serving.

85.Grilled Peaches with Coconut Cream

Serves: 12

Ingredients:

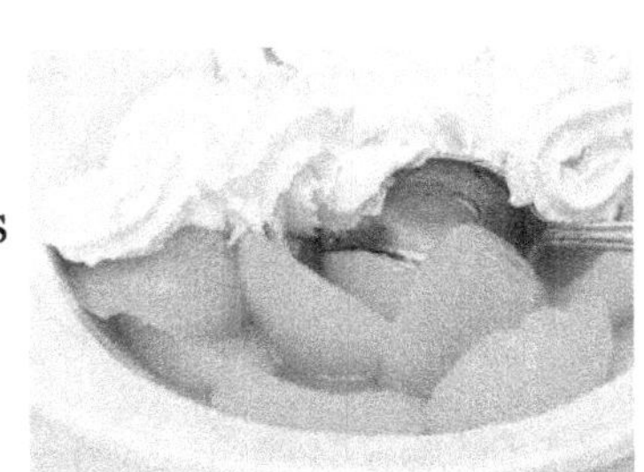

- 6 medium ripe peaches, halved, pitted,
- 2 cans coconut milk, chilled for 8-10 hours
- ½ tsp ground cinnamon or to taste
- ½ cup chopped, walnuts
- 2 tsp vanilla extract
- Stevia drops or swerve sweetener to taste (optional)

Method:

1. Coconut cream will be on the top of the cans of coconut milk. Remove the cream from it and add into a bowl. Use the remaining coconut milk for some other recipe like in a smoothie or curry.
2. Add vanilla into the bowl of coconut cream and beat well with an electric hand mixer. Add sweetener while beating if using.
3. Place the peaches on a preheated grill with the cut side facing down on the grill. Grill for 3-4 minutes. Flip sides and grill for 3-4 minutes.
4. Place 1 piece of peach in each bowl.
5. Spoon the coconut cream over it. Sprinkle cinnamon and walnuts on top and serve.

86. Chocolate Coconut Cream Mousse

Serves: 4

Ingredients:

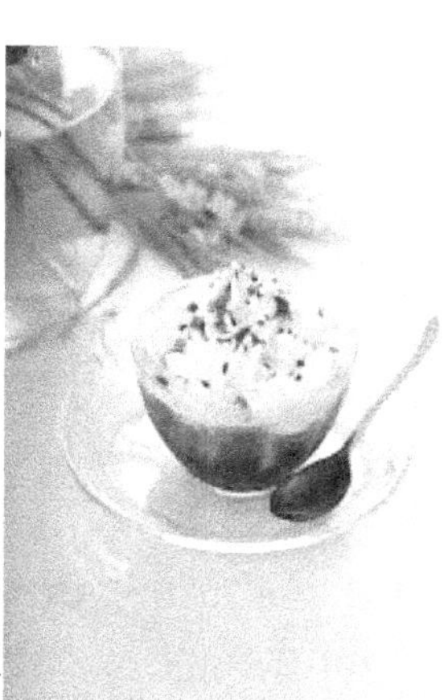

- 2 cans (14.5 ounces each) full fat coconut milk, chilled for 4-5 hours
- 4 tbsp swerve or erythritol or to taste
- 4 tsp vanilla extract
- 4 tbsp cocoa, unsweetened
- Cocoa nibs, to garnish

Method:

1. Remove the coconut cream that is floating on the top with a spoon and add into a mixing bowl. Use the liquid remaining in the can for some other recipe like in a smooth.
2. Add rest of the ingredients and whip well.
3. Spoon into bowls. Chill for a while and serve garnished with cocoa nibs.

87. Raw Brownie Bites

Serves: 12-15

Ingredients:

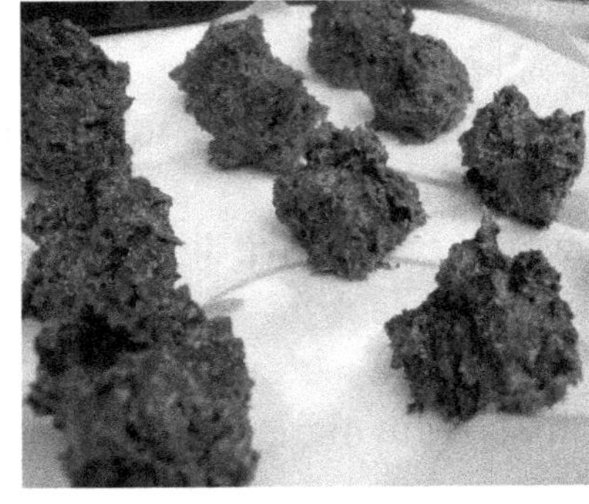

- 3 cups walnuts
- 2 cups pitted dates
- 2/3 cup cocoa powder
- A pinch salt
- 2 tsp vanilla extract

Method:

1. Add walnuts and salt into the food processor bowl. Pulse until finely ground.
2. Add rest of the ingredients and process until fine. Add 1-2 tbsp water through the feeder tube and pulse until the mixture comes together.
3. Transfer into a bowl. Make small balls of the mixture using your hands. Place in an airtight container.
4. It can last for a week in the refrigerator.

88. Orange Creamsicles

Serves: 5

Ingredients:

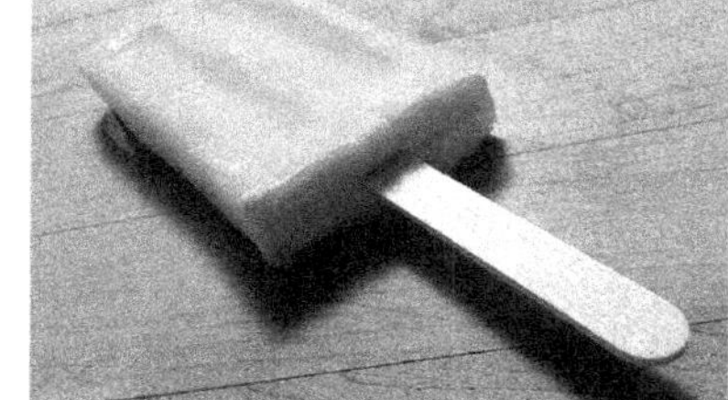

- ¾ cup almond milk, unsweetened
- ¾ cup fresh orange juice, unsweetened

Method

1. Add orange juice and almond milk into a bowl. Whisk until well combined.
2. Pour into Popsicle molds. Insert the Popsicle sticks.
3. Freeze until firm.
4. Pour some hot water on the bottom of the mold to loosen.
5. Remove from the Popsicle mold and serve.

89. Strawberry Banana Cheesecake

Serves: 16

Ingredients:

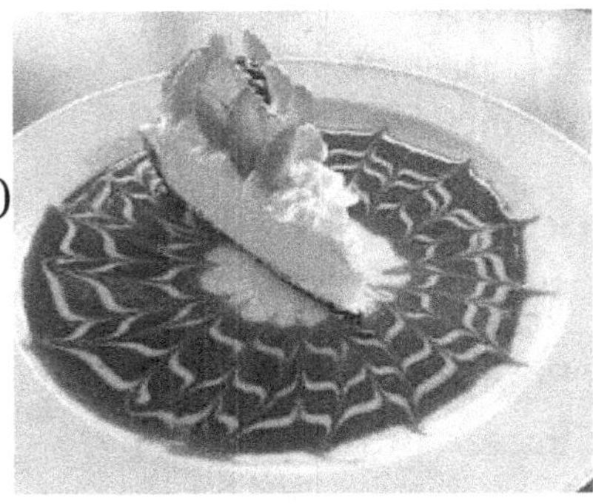

- 3 cups almond flour
- 4 cups strawberry puree
- 7 ounces solid creamed coconut (Santen) chopped into small pieces
- 2 tbsp arrowroot powder
- ½ cup coconut oil, melted
- 4 large bananas, sliced
- 6 eggs
- ½ tsp vanilla powder

Method:

1. Add oil and almond flour into a bowl and mix using your hands to get crumbs.
2. Transfer into a large quiche pan or tart pan or use 2 smaller pans. Press it well onto the bottom of the pan.
3. Add rest of the ingredients into a blender and blend until smooth. Pour over the crust in the pan.
4. Bake in a preheated oven at 350 ° F for about 35-40 minutes or until set.
5. Cool completely and refrigerate until it is very chilled.
6. Slice and serve chilled.

90. Popsicle Treats

Serves: 8

Ingredients:

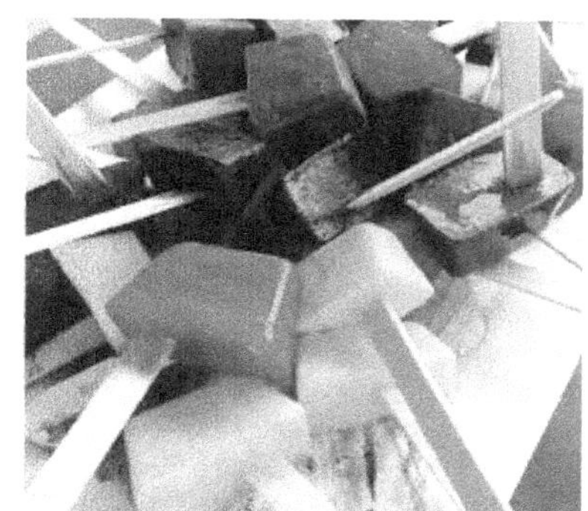

- 8 slices kiwi fruit
- ½ cup blueberries
- 8 grapes, halved
- 8 slices strawberries
- 8 slices melon
- Coconut water, as required

Method:

1. Place a slice of kiwi, strawberry and melon in each of 8 Popsicle molds.
2. Place 2 grape halves in each mold.
3. Divide and add the blueberries into the molds.
4. Fill the molds with coconut water. Do not fill right up to the top.
5. Insert the Popsicle sticks in it.
6. Freeze until firm.
7. Pour some hot water on the bottom of the mold to loosen.
8. Remove from the Popsicle mold and serve.

Conclusion

Thank you once again for choosing this book and I hope you found it useful and informative.

Intermittent fasting is one of the best ways to lose weight without making your body or mind suffer. Although it may sound and seem difficult in the beginning, with proper support and resources, you can become an intermittent faster in no time.

This book tackled one of the major myths about intermittent fasting - that you cannot eat or drink anything interesting while you practice intermittent fasting. All the recipes come with special instructions and details steps so you can never go wrong with them. Just keep an eye on ingredients and portions and you are good to go. You will definitely lose weight without craving all the time thanks to these recipes.

Now that you have all the recipes that you need to begin an intermittent fast, why wait? Get in the kitchen and start cooking!

Good luck!

Don't Forget your Free Book!

As a token of appreciation for you purchasing my book, I would like to give you a **<u>free book</u>**!

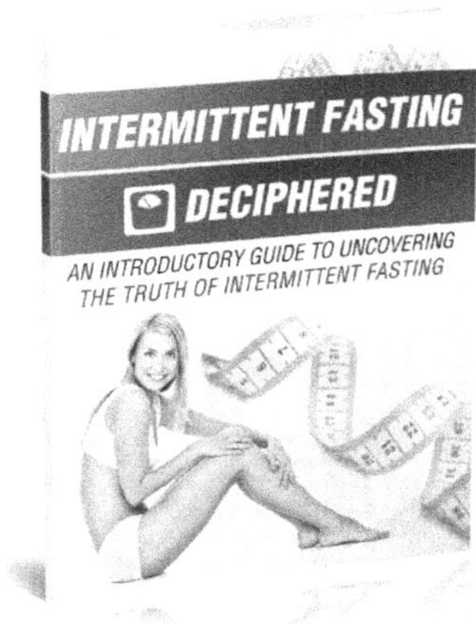

You can get you book by clicking here: (or type it into your browser if you are reading the paperback)

https://bit.ly/2MbQ3vE

www.ingramcontent.com/pod-product-compliance
Lightning Source LLC
Chambersburg PA
CBHW081620250726
48657CB00009B/2638